CARTELS
AT
WAR

Related Titles from Potomac Books

Drugs and Contemporary Warfare
—Paul Rexton Kan

Axis of Unity: Venezuela, Iran & the Threat to America
—Sean Goforth

*The War of All the People: The Nexus of Latin American Radicalism
and Middle Eastern Terrorism*
—Jon B. Perdue

Mexico's Drug-Fueled Violence and the Threat to U.S. National Security

CARTELS
AT
WAR

PAUL REXTON KAN
FOREWORD BY GEN. BARRY R. McCAFFREY, USA (RET.)

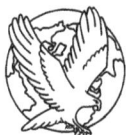

Potomac Books
Washington, D.C.

Library of Congress Cataloging-in-Publication Data
Kan, Paul Rexton.
    Cartels at war : Mexico's drug-fueled violence and the threat to U.S. national security / Paul Rexton Kan ; foreword by Barry R. McCaffrey.—1st ed.
        p. cm.
    Includes bibliographical references and index.
    ISBN 978-1-59797-707-4 (hbk. : alk. paper)—ISBN 978-1-59797-805-7 (electronic)
    1. Drug traffic—Mexico. 2. Drug control—Mexico. 3. Narco-terrorism—Mexico.
    4. Violent crimes—Mexico. 5. Organized crime—Mexico. 6. Refugees—Mexico.
    7. National security—United States. 8. United States—Emigration and immigration—
    Government policy. I. Title.
        HV5840.M4K36 2012
        363.450972—dc23
                                                                                    2012027665

Printed in the United States of America on acid-free paper that meets the American National Standards Institute Z39-48 Standard.

Potomac Books
22841 Quicksilver Drive
Dulles, Virginia 20166

First Edition

CONTENTS

FOREWORD

Paul Kan has produced a magnificent analysis and equally thoughtful policy recommendations to deal with the dreadful situation faced by our giant Mexican
southern neighbor as they face a bloody and complex internal struggle to establish
the rule of law in the face of the enormously violent drug cartels. We should be
grateful that Paul Kan has been supported and guided by the faculty of the U.S.
Army War College at Carlisle, Pennsylvania, where he holds the Henry L. Stimson
Chair of Military Studies. His first book, *Drugs and Contemporary Warfare*, and
his many articles on the intersection of drug trafficking, crime, and modern forms
of armed conflict have made him the leading national expert on a new type of
asymmetric warfare that now challenges the capabilities of our law enforcement,
intelligence, and military establishments. This brilliant book is now the definitive
work available to understand the ferocious struggle for the soul of Mexico currently taking place among the 113 million Mexicans who live south of our two-
thousand-mile common border.

The internal threat to Mexican institutions approximates the conditions of general warfare as these armed criminal gangs compete with the state for power. To date,
53,000 Mexicans have been murdered. Cartel gangs employ .50-caliber anti-aircraft
guns, rocket-propelled grenades, military hand grenades, armored vehicles, helicop-
ters, submarines, signals intelligence intercept equipment, information warfare, and
automatic weapons by the thousands to completely dominate local police, and corrupt and intimidate state and federal police. The cartels will also engage in direct and
open warfare against Mexican marines and the army. This battle for control of
Mexico's future is not confined to the toxic U.S.-Mexico border states. Half the states
of Mexico are now in contention. The business capital of Monterrey and the lush
resorts of the tourist areas are no longer assured of security by Mexican law enforcement. You can be murdered if you are a Catholic cardinal, a Mexican army general,

the leading presidential candidate, a journalist, or a young girl trying to make a living wage to send home to your mother while working in a border maquiladora.

The former Mexican PAN party administration of President Calderón displayed enormous courage and organizational skill to confront these malignant criminal groups. Fortunately it is hard to imagine Mexico becoming a failed state only because of the loyalty and monopoly of legitimate and overwhelming power that the Mexican armed forces can assemble at any given point on this dangerous battlefield. These cartel gangs do not fight for ideology—they compete for billions of dollars of criminal profits. They welcome chaos and fear. They have created impunity to the law. There is also a clear element of mindless cruelty and nihilism to this struggle. The slaughter of innocent migrant Central Americans and the depraved torture of civilians open a dark window into the cultural forces at play here. The pragmatic cartel mafia business leaders are now dead, extradited to the United States, or in hiding. The killers and psychopaths are now in charge of the criminal groups.

The United States has failed to realistically engage our vital national security interests in concert with the Mexican government. We owe Mexico a better level of cooperation. We know a strategy requires both a conceptual framework for action and the resources to implement the plan. In dealing with Mexico's internal threat we have neither. The Mérida Initiative is an anemic attempt to support a Mexican government struggling for the survival of democracy—$1.3 billion in U.S. funding for a multiyear Mérida effort compares unfavorably to the $10 billion a month we currently burn in Afghanistan. Mexico and Canada as the NAFTA cooperative states are clearly the two dominant economic, criminal justice, cultural, diplomatic, and national security partners of the United States. The political energy and resources we devote to these vital U.S. interests are, at face value, inadequate.

Historically we should take note that our support of Colombia during the Clinton and George W. Bush administrations with Plan Colombia gave Bogota the basic tools (combined with the courage and leadership of the Urribe and Santos administrations) to break the back of the FARC, the National Liberation Party, and the United Self-Defense Forces of Colombia. No such level of support has been organized for our vital Mexican partner. We the United States are in denial. The cartel violence has crossed our border and threatens U.S. security. Mexican cartels are now the dominant organized crime activity in over two hundred American cities. The cartel foot soldiers are recruited in the U.S. prison system among the 2.1 million we hold behind bars in local, state, and federal incarceration. The cartels now dominate the wholesale smuggling and distribution of methamphetamines, high THC–content pot, ecstasy pills, and Colombian cocaine. Mexican grown and

refined heroin supplies as much as half of the U.S. consumption. These Mexican cartels do immensely more damage to our citizens than either the Taliban or al Qaeda.
They are now expanding into new criminal enterprises of exploitation of women,
home invasions, firearms violations, money laundering, extortion, and kidnapping
and murder of U.S. citizens as well as Mexican illegal immigrants.

The central challenge to Mexico is not to break the cartels with military power.
Their crucial challenge is to build a system of justice that allows and can impose
the rule of law. This means not just the creation of a Mexican federal police force
of integrity, competence, training, technology, and values that can withstand the
horrible threat of the gangs. The justice system clearly also requires judicial courts
that can function with security and integrity—and prosecutors with the institutional armor to withstand personal danger and bribes to enforce the rule of law.
Finally, nothing will happen unless there is an expectation that legal, court-imposed
punishment can happen. The Mexican prison system is a cesspool of criminality
and a revolving door for the dangerous cartel gangs that self-administer themselves
behind bars. Simply stated, there is no justice in Mexico. The most violent and
shocking of cartel felonies have only a 1 percent chance of arrest, prosecution, and
punishment. The bottom line is that it is much more difficult to build a system of
justice than a competent and disciplined military fighting force.

Paul Kan has done a thoroughly commendable analytical job of objective scholar-
ship with this book. This is the single best work available for a thoughtful understanding of the challenges we face in Mexico. We must act. There is a significant
possibility that the next Mexican administration led by the PRI after two reformists
administrations of the PAN party will conclude that the burdens of this struggle are
not bearable. The next Mexican president could consider an accommodation with
these terrible narco-criminals. Minus the courage and resistance of Mexican authorities that we have seen during the Calderón administration, we would face chaos south
of our border. The Mexican people would be lost for a generation.

Paul Kan has given us the conceptual framework to understand this challenge. It
is time to turn our attention south. Mexico is vital to our future. They are a people of
tremendous dedication to hard work, spirituality, humility, and generosity. The culture and the energy of Mexico have deeply and positively affected the United States.
Now is the time to act with a level of support and leadership commensurate with the
importance of these beautiful people to the future of North America.

Gen. Barry R. McCaffrey, USA (Ret.)
former director, National Drug Policy, 1996–2001

PREFACE

I was researching another book when the editor of my previous book, Hilary Claggett, contacted me and suggested that the topic of Mexico needed some coverage. She asked me whether I would be interested in submitting a book proposal. I thought surely someone else had already published a book about Mexico's drug-fueled violence. Upon further investigation and research, I did find a number of books that examined the issue, so what would be my contribution to the outstanding existing literature on the subject?

I later remembered that in the course of an interview with a detective from the drug enforcement task force in my county for the book project I had been previously working on, he casually mentioned that two gang members with links to the Juarez cartel were caught at a local motel. I remember being dumbfounded. The motel is only three miles from my house. Plus, I work at the U.S. Army War College, whose students are engaged in fighting two wars overseas, but here was a threat that was literally very close to home.

When I mentioned to my department chairperson that I was considering some research along the Mexican border, he told me that I'd better come back with all my body parts in their current arrangement. In another instance, a close friend of mine mentioned that she was doing some work around her house and had the TV news on in the background. When she looked at the scenes of violence in Afghanistan, she wondered why all the witnesses were speaking in Spanish. Then she realized her mistake—the report was about a gun battle that killed twenty-one people twelve miles south of the U.S. border.

Amid all these conversations, I found questions that needed to be answered for many people, including myself. This book is a small contribution to that quest, to understanding why Mexico has become so violent and why those of us in the United States should care. It is written from an American perspective with a deep appreciation of the country of Mexico. I worked and volunteered in orphanages in Tijuana and Tecate as a college student; I also worked in bilingual high school classrooms as a graduate student in Denver. I have only known the gracious side of that country and its people, a side that is now increasingly being overshadowed by such terrible acts of violence that many policymakers and scholars suggest it will become a failed state.

There is no doubt that failure of the Mexican state would be of vital concern to the United States. In many ways, this book is written from a speculative vantage point looking backward—if Mexico failed, how would we explain what caused it, and what could the United States have done to prevent it? I would argue that Mexico was a victim of high-intensity crime brought about by cartels at war and that the United States was caught largely unprepared.

Many have looked to the history and politics of Mexico or have spoken to Americans' demand to be supplied with intoxicating narcotics as explanations. Others have traveled the length of the border between the two countries or spent time in some of the most dangerous Mexican cities to provide clues that explain the enduring violence that has become a spectacle. All of them have helped inform this work. But what I am doing is to talk about the situation in Mexico as a war, but not one that is familiar to a good deal of scholars, decision makers, military officials, or the general public. The violence might seem the same, as do the effects on neighboring states as well as the daily struggle of those innocents caught in the maelstrom of uncertainty and potential death. It is a multidimensional, multiparty, multilocation conflict fought over criminal goals—a mosaic cartel war. And coming to grips with it will mean using multiple differing perspectives to inform as many audiences as possible. This book is only one perspective.

My previous book, *Drugs and Contemporary Warfare*, examined how warring groups like guerrillas, insurgents, terrorists, and professional militaries were trafficking drugs in order to keep themselves viable in the aftermath of the Cold War. This book's thesis is nearly the reverse—how drug cartels in Mexico are warring in order to keep their profits flowing. It wasn't an easy pivot to make, and any mistakes as a result are purely my own.

It is my hope that scholars and policymakers will find this book as an additional point of view. Policymakers may find the book as a way to thicken the ongoing discussions and debates. Those who are concerned with Mexico as a general interest, whom scholars and policymakers all serve in one way or another, may gravitate toward my thesis because it easy to grasp and begins a conversation of what can be done in the here and now.

ACKNOWLEDGMENTS

I have heard many scholars and colleagues say that the first book is the hardest. I wondered, "What makes the second book easier?!" The answer is found in all the efforts and support of the following people. At my professional home of the U.S. Army War College, I have been very fortunate to be colleagues with first-rate minds like Tony Echevarria, Jim Helis, and Frank Jones, who have supported my efforts and nudged my work (and my prose) in better directions than I could've found on my own. Our college's commandant, Maj. Gen. Gregg Martin, has been very supportive of my work and to new ways of thinking. Phil Williams of the University of Pittsburgh has been a great mentor for me from the time he was a visiting scholar at the War College through today. The administrative support from BJ Saylor, John Winegardner, Matt Bittle, and Tara Colyer is something that I will never forget (not that they would allow me to forget it). Jeanette Moyer and Nancy Sneed at the Army War College Library were very patient with my repeated requests for obscure sources while sending me helpful sources that came their way. The maps and graphs were done with the assistance of Dave Buceta in the Army War College Graphics Department. I have also had the benefit of working with some top-notch interns from Dickinson College—Dan Owins, Nick Iorio, and Brett Lerner—who ran down some critical research for this book.

To those outside the Army War College community, I also owe thanks to Diego Valle-Jones at his eclectic website, blog.diegovalle.net, for assisting me with a variety of statistical analyses and to Christopher Albon at www.conflicthealth.com for allowing me to post a few entries on this topic on his blog as a way to test out this book's thesis.

The professional expertise of those in the policy and law enforcement realms were extremely valuable in helping ensure that my ivory tower pursuits met the real world of drug trafficking. From among them, I owe a special debt to Carl

Landrum of the U.S. Border Patrol, who was one of my students at the Army War College but who has been my mentor as I entered the world of Mexican cartel operations that he works in every day. My gratitude also extends to Joseph Ralph, Michael Hayes, and Roberto Del Villar of the U.S. Border Patrol; Gil Kerlikowske, Pat Ward, and Brad Hittle of the Office of National Drug Control Policy; Matt Stoffolano of the National Park Service; and Tom Schultz of the FBI. I would also like to thank ranchers Warner Glenn and Kelly Kimbro.

It was a real pleasure to work again with the folks at Potomac Books, especially Hilary Claggett and Claire Noble.

For their friendship and moral support, Chrisi Arrighi, Chris Mescow, Alison Zapata, Shawn Morris, Troy Gagliano, Erica Briggs, Kevin Rockwood, Michael Powers, Lou Dejoie, the Nunez family.

Finally, I am especially thankful for my family—Elwyn Kan, Monique Kan-Souza, Kevin Souza, Janae Souza, and Kiani Souza—who continue to keep my personal and professional life on the right track.

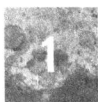

THE OUTBREAK
The Wars Begin

In 2009, John Cook, mayor of El Paso, Texas, expressed his bewilderment: "It's strange to be the third-safest city in the United States right next to a war zone."[1] The "war zone" the mayor referred to is across the border in Ciudad Juarez, Mexico, where over 6,000 people have been killed since 2006. In 2010, there was one homicide in El Paso. In that same year in Juarez, someone was slain every three hours.[2] The city became so dangerous in 2010 that the U.S. Department of State encouraged nonessential consulate workers to return to the United States after two American employees were targeted and killed by a local drug gang. Since 2006, over 50,000 Mexicans have been killed, and many Mexican cities have witnessed horrific scenes of drug cartel cruelty, including dismemberment and beheadings. By 2008, there were more beheadings occurring in Mexico than in Iraq and Afghanistan combined. And outside of these two war-torn countries, Mexico has become the place where more Americans have been killed than any other nation, most victims of cartel violence.[3] This has all occurred in the shadow of 50,000 Mexican army troops, deployed on the streets of several cities to control the violence after local, state, and federal law enforcement agencies failed.

Communities in the United States have not been immune from this violence. Home invasions have surged in Phoenix, Arizona, and kidnappings exceeded one a day in 2008 as Mexican street gangs sought to enforce agreements or settle grudges from cartel wars in Mexico. In the spring of 2010, Sheriff Arvin West told residents of his border county of Hudspeth, Texas, to arm themselves because he could no longer protect them from the spillover of violence occurring in the Juarez Valley of Mexico. He exclaimed at a town hall meeting, "You farmers, I'm telling you right now, arm yourselves. As they say the old story is, it's better to be tried by twelve than carried by six. Damn it, I don't want to see six people carrying you!"[4] A cartel member is wanted in the killing of a Dallas police officer,[5] and armed gang

1

members routinely cross the U.S.-Mexico border to protect drug shipments into the United States.[6]

But the spillover of cartel violence is only one of the effects that demonstrate the perilous situation in Mexico. Since 2006, there has been a rise in the number of Mexican nationals seeking political asylum in the United States to escape the ongoing drug cartel violence in their home country. In 2011, 5,000 Mexicans lodged formal asylum requests in the United States, representing a 168 percent increase over the year before.[7] Although the numbers appear small, it is the sudden jump in requests in such a short span of time that is concerning. In 2006, just as Mexican president Felipe Calderón declared war on the cartels, only fifty-four Mexicans sought asylum, and no Mexicans asked for asylum in the 1990s during that decade's brief but bloody outbreak of drug cartel violence.[8] Those who are being targeted by cartels and gangs are police who investigate crimes, mayors who govern towns, journalists who write about the violence, and ordinary citizens who are in the way. If criminal violence continues, increases, or spreads, U.S. communities will feel an even greater burden on their systems of public safety and public health from "narco-refugees."

Mexican drug violence has set off alarm bells for those who work in the corridors of U.S. national security. After a visit to Mexico in late 2008, for example, Gen. Barry McCaffrey, former head of the U.S. Office of National Drug Control Policy, wrote that:

A failure by the Mexican political system to curtail lawlessness and violence could result in a surge of millions of refugees crossing the U.S. border to escape domestic misery of violence, failed economic policy, poverty, hunger, joblessness, and the mindless cruelty and injustice of a criminal state. Mexico is not confronting dangerous criminality—it is fighting for survival against narcoterrorism.[9]

Indeed, one of the first stops for the incoming Obama administration's national security team was Mexico. The president himself was also pressed into commenting on the conditions that might bring a more forceful U.S. response to the violence: "I think it's unacceptable if you've got drug gangs crossing our borders and killing U.S. citizens. I think if one U.S. citizen is killed because of foreign nationals who are engaging in violent crime, that's enough of a concern to do something about it."[10]

Doing something about the violence is exceptionally thorny. There is a mutually reinforcing dynamic that is fueling the violence in Mexico that is spilling into the United States. The limited amount of economic opportunity in Mexico and the compromised nature of its political system have created a ripe environment for drug cartels and gangs to take advantage of Americans' long-standing desire for illicit narcotics. Americans spend between $18 billion and $39 billion annually on narcotics coming northward.[11] As former Mexican attorney general Eduardo Medina Mora stated, "In that sense, the United States is already financing this war. It is just financing the wrong side."[12] Drug profits outstrip many areas of the legitimate commerce between the two nations; annual remittances going southbound from the Mexican community in the United States total $23 billion,[13] and the revenues generated by the Mexican tourism industry before the recession totaled nearly $11 billion.[14] The power of the clandestine economy has also undermined Mexico's governmental institutions. Only 5 percent of crimes in the country are solved,[15] while only 1 to 2 percent lead to conviction or jail time.[16] This has created "zones of impunity" described by President Calderón where several Mexican cities have allowed cartels to operate freely and to continue supplying America with narcotics while profits have been used to further challenge the power of the Mexican state and to undermine civil society.

A symbiotic relationship has emerged between weak governance on one hand and strong drug consumption on the other. As such, the U.S.-Mexico border runs along the nexus of national security and public safety. Yet managing this nexus will require that policymakers respond with carefully calibrated approaches to prevent stoking more cartel violence, increasing the incentives to smuggle drugs into the United States, and eroding Mexican governmental capacity. Because of the complexity of the violence and its effects, this book uses insights from a number of disciplines— history, political science, sociology, criminology, economics, and international relations—to provide a greater understanding of the ongoing cartel war in Mexico and to develop appropriate approaches that would bring it to a conclusion.

Structural Causes of Mexico's Cartel War

Several factors and events led to the recent outbreak of the Mexican cartel war. The North American Free Trade Agreement (NAFTA), signed in 1994 by the United States, Canada, and Mexico, created the world's largest trading block by removing tariffs on trade and investment among the three nations. While removing barriers made access to each market easier for licit flows of goods, it also did the same for illicit businesses. Phil Jordan was the Drug Enforcement Administration's (DEA) director of the El Paso Intelligence Center during the early implementation of NAFTA and described the trade agreement as a "deal made in narco-heaven."[17]

4 CARTELS AT WAR

For Mexican drug cartels, the provisions of NAFTA came at an opportune time, when U.S. interdiction of Colombian cocaine in the Caribbean was increasingly taxing Colombian groups while the demand for methamphetamine in the United States skyrocketed. Mexican cartels were able to capitalize on newly available overland routes to bring cocaine and meth to the U.S. market. The first year of NAFTA's implementation there was a 25 percent rise in commercial-vehicle smuggling cases—the biggest jump on record.[18] In addition, the number of meth-related emergency room visits in the United States doubled between 1991 and 1994.[19]

NAFTA as a boon to cartels created the conditions for the first spasm of drug-fueled violence in Mexico. Cartels fought among each other, and they often directed their violent campaigns against the government and civil society, all for control of new cargo, routes, and territory. Mexico was wracked by a high caliber of drug violence in the early 1990s, such as the killing of Cardinal Ocampo at Guadalajara Airport in 1993 and the assassination of the Partido Revolucionario Institucional (PRI) presidential candidate Luis Donaldo Colosio in 1994. Six years later, a federal prosecutor, his two aides, a special prosecutor, and a Mexican army captain were killed in the span of one month; their bodies were found with almost every bone broken, "like a sack of ice cubes," and their heads were crushed by an industrial press.[20]

The loss of political power by the PRI in Mexico also contributed to Mexican cartel wars of the 1990s and to the ongoing cartel war of today. Drug traffickers in Mexico historically required the permission of governors along with the collusion of the military and police to operate.[21] For the majority of the twentieth century, the PRI acted as a referee and market enforcer among various drug smuggling groups that lent relative stability to the trade in illicit narcotics. "The cartels provided bribes and kept violence to a minimum. In return, the PRI protected the kingpins and resolved conflicts between them, most notably by allocating access to the drug corridors (*plazas*) to the United States."[22] During the late 1980s and into the 1990s, however, these traditional arrangements began to break down as the PRI became weaker while new opportunities for trafficking cocaine and meth rose for Mexican drug trafficking organizations. "Electoral competition nullified the unwritten understandings, requiring drug lords to negotiate with the new political establishment and encouraging rival traffickers to bid for new market opportunities."[23] This represented a shift in the balance of power within what Roy Godson termed the political-criminal nexus, resulting in a violent free-for-all as criminal organizations seized new opportunities, attempted to establish territorial dominance over the plazas, and competed for a greater share of illicit markets.[24]

The definitive disintegration of the political-criminal nexus occurred when the PRI lost the presidency in both 2000 and 2006 to the right-leaning Partido Accion Nacional (PAN).Both successive governments took a more confrontational stance toward Mexican drug trafficking organizations. PAN's first president, Vicente Fox, briefly sent the Mexican army to two cities along the U.S. border to tackle the cartels and promised to fight "the mother of all battles" against them.[25] Part of the reason for this confrontation was the side effects of the terrorist attacks of 9/11 that renewed U.S. attention to border security and placed greater focus on border crossings from familiar plazas. Increased focus on U.S. ports of entry and well-traveled smuggling routes forced cartels to compete over alternative routes, while cartels and gangs competed to find ways to compensate for this loss of income. They did so by stimulating a consumer market at home; the cartels began selling drugs in Mexico. Once again, this broke a tacit understanding with the previous PRI government. There had been "an unspoken agreement with the government that gangs would be tolerated as long as they didn't sell the drugs in Mexico but passed them on instead to the gringos. Since 2001, local demand for cocaine has grown an estimated 20 percent per year."[26] Not only did this force Fox's hand, but the cartels and gangs sought to carve out new areas in local markets, leading to more conflict and violence that the government sought to contain.

But it was Felipe Calderón's razor-thin election to the presidency in 2006 that created the spark for the current cartel wars. After winning by a narrow margin of 0.58 percentage points, Calderón chose a platform to increase his legitimacy among Mexicans after weeks of demonstrations by supporters of his opponents and amid accusations of electoral fraud. Ten days after his inauguration on December 1, 2006, Calderón sent 6,500 military personnel to a number of the most violent Mexican cities and declared war on drug cartels. "The most important reason for the December 11, 2006, declaration of war was political: to achieve legitimacy supposedly lost at the ballot box."[27] Calderón's decision to take a more confrontational response, however, can also be viewed as a consequence of NAFTA. The burgeoning Mexican middle class is the product of increased economic opportunities in the hemisphere; large segments of this class have demanded public transparency, judicial reform, and, most of all, safety. As a member of this growing middle class, Calderón was responding to these voters who gave him his narrow electoral win.[28]

Some of the killings of agents of the state are in retaliation for the PAN's interference in the drug trafficking business. In effect, the violence is the cost the administrations of Vicente Fox and Felipe Calderón have had to pay for defecting from the tacit acquiescence that characterized successive PRI governments. In some instances, cartels have intentionally increased the insecurity of ordinary Mexicans as a signal to the government to back off its current strategy to bring down the cartels.

All of these factors and events—the signing of NAFTA, the end of PRI political dominance, greater PAN confrontation of cartels, and changes in the patterns of drug trafficking—helped the cartels evolve into the current violent menaces to the Mexican state that they are today. New trafficking opportunities combined with better enforcement meant that cartels required "deep pockets to run sophisticated logistics needed to escape detection and seizure, pay the necessary bribes, and absorb substantial losses of their product when seizures happen. These barriers to entry have winnowed the trafficking business down to a handful of major players."[29] In fact, the Mexican cartel wars of the 1990s left behind many "veterans" who now seek revenge for acts committed years ago while new members now seek to prove themselves by participating in these feuds. By 2006, drug traffickers coalesced into seven major cartels that now control 90 percent of the illicit narcotics imports into the United States.[30] These major players are the actors largely responsible for inflicting the ongoing and bloody violence upon Mexican society, defying many familiar terms and concepts associated with large-scale death at the hands of armed groups operating in the shadow of the state.

Not Insurgency, Not Terrorism, and Not a Crime Wave

There has been a very active debate over how to describe the violence that is occurring in Mexico. Is it narco-insurgency, narco-terrorism, or a crime wave that is gripping Mexico? This is more than a mere academic debate; labeling the violence is important to understanding how its eruption began, its dynamics, and the strategies to bring it to an end. Such distinctions may not seem important as all insurgent groups, terrorist organizations, and organized crime syndicates share a number of organizational and operational characteristics.

They (1) are involved in illegal activities and frequently need the same supplies; (2) exploit excessive violence and the threat of violence; (3) commit kidnappings, assassinations and extortion; (4) act in secrecy; (5) challenge the state and the laws (unless they are state funded); (6) have back up leaders and foot soldiers; (7) are exceedingly adaptable, open to innovations, and are flexible; (8) threaten global security; (9) enact deadly consequences for former members who have quit the group.[31]

However, defining what sort of organized violence is happening has deep and far reaching implications for policymakers who design strategies that eventually must be implemented by those who face the effects of the ongoing violence on a daily basis. Terms like insurgency and terrorism create policy options and strategic choices that are different from those that would be responses to criminality.

Several scholars and commentators not only agree with Barry McCaffrey's assertion that Mexico is experiencing narco-terrorism but go even farther. Hal Brands has called Mexican violence a "multisided narco-insurgency; well-financed cartels are doing battle with the government and one another for control of the drug corridors into the United States . . . significantly destabilizing internal order in Mexico."[32] Secretary of State Hillary Clinton described Mexico as "looking more and more like Colombia looked twenty years ago."[33] The cartels are able to destabilize Mexico because they "have better weapons and better armor than Mexican or U.S. law enforcement. They have similar, and often superior, training."[34] They are, simply put, "the guerrillas next door."[35] Luis Astorga, a sociologist at the Institute of Social Research in Mexico City, laments that "right now it's not very clear what the 'war' means. No one is sure who is fighting who. It best resembles a circular firing squad."[36] For Robert Bunker, the result is a "state that is no longer able to govern entire sectors within its sovereign territory, and instead, these areas have been taken over by a narco-insurgency and lost to the influence of criminal-based entities."[37] Mexicans generally call it "La Inseguridad"—the insecurity. The implications, according to Max Manwaring, may be "some manifestation of state failure."[38]

Given the targets, scope, intensity, and effects of the violence, it is tempting to agree with notions that Mexico is experiencing a type of intrastate war or a direct assault against the state. However, if the arguments of the narco-insurgency/narco-terrorism school are accurate in describing the situation in Mexico, they must answer a number of questions, which so far have been troublesome. The first set of questions surround why the violence began. If cartels are akin to insurgents or terrorists, what are their grievances, and what political or social goals are they fighting to achieve to assuage these grievances? In short, what is the "rallying cry" for their constituency? As discussed in the previous section, the current outbreak of cartel violence is a continuation of the Mexican cartel wars of the 1990s that were primarily motivated by new trafficking opportunities, the breakdown in the political-criminal nexus, and improved border security. The successes that cartels have had in penetrating the political realm of Mexico or purging local communities of mayors and police through bribery, extortion, and coercive violence have been to ensure the smooth operation of cartel profit-making activities in the illicit drug trade. In these instances, they have not "captured" the state to implement a social or political agenda, but have sought to get the state out of the way. For example, according to the trial testimony of former Juarez police captain Manuel Fierro-Mendez, cartels seek to control plazas "to maintain order over the local, state, and federal agencies then to have free reign to continue trafficking drugs without any problem."[39] Terror and insurgent groups have constituents that they are trying to sway with their violence, while cartels have clients for their product and services that they are attempting to satisfy by circumventing or undermining the state.[40] Unlike terrorists and insurgents, the cartels in Mexico are not motivated to create a homeland to call their own, substitute their ideology for the existing one, or to achieve any other sort of political goal that is routinely associated with armed groups who instigate social upheaval.

Another critical question is whether tactical qualities of the cartels equal an insurgent or terrorist threat to the Mexican state. The narco-insurgency/narco-terrorism school argues that they do because of the cartels sophisticated weaponry and the proficiency of their violence often match or outstrip the police and military. But equipment and tactics do not exist in isolation. Improved tactics, skills, and weaponry of cartels are not a substitute for a strategic political objective that tactics are intended to serve. Having better weapons does not compensate for a cause. It would be as if J. Edgar Hoover declared Al Capone and his gang to be insurgents because they had tommy guns while local police merely had pistols. Another related question is who are the targets of cartel violence? The answer is revealing—less than 10 percent of the deaths in Mexico have been agents of the state. If there were an all-out assault by the cartels against the Mexican state, as in an insurgency, the proportion would be much higher. Even violent acts by the cartels and gangs that have been directed at government targets are meant to signal the government to retreat from its confrontational stance; they are to intimidate the government rather than to serve as a political statement.[41] In fact, the violence directed at the state mirrors the levels and types of violence that were used by Colombia's Medellin cartel in the 1980s when Pablo Escobar directed attacks against the Palace of Justice and was responsible for the mid-air destruction of a passenger jet, killing 110 people. Like the Medellin cartel, Mexican cartels seek to intimidate the state to protect their economic interests, keep themselves out of jail, and remove their families from harm's way.[42] The fact that the narco-insurgency/narco-terrorism school focuses the bulk of its attention on cartel violence against the state misses the importance of the vast majority of violence happening between and within cartels themselves. Such a lack of attention and analysis forms a large gap in its overall analysis of what is happening in Mexico.

The strategic reasons for violence and the tactics employed by the cartels do not suggest that the narco-insurgency/narco-terrorism school is accurate in its assessment of the situation in Mexico; addressing questions about how to end the violence also weakens its analysis. Most insurgent and terrorist groups have goals that are negotiable, once again because these goals are generally political in nature. Because the violence in Mexico is not low-intensity conflict, any sort of negotiations with the cartels in Mexico would take different contours. The criminal nature of their enterprise would forestall the willingness of the government or cartels to find the common ground needed to begin a "peace process" that would lead to the disarmament, demobilization, and reintegration of cartel and gang members. Would the Mexican government grant pardons and amnesties for cartel leaders and gang members if they agree to no longer traffic narcotics? Such an offer, implausible as it is, would unlikely be accepted by a cartel whose main motivation is making money through illicit activities; it would be an invitation to go out of business. However, negotiations to reduce violence in exchange for continuing to traffic drugs may be plausible. Even if the previous arrangements under the PRI were somehow reconstituted as a way to end or reduce the violence, this would once again reveal the fundamental economic and financial nature, rather than the political nature, of the cartels' motivations.

Outside of successful peace negotiations, terrorism and insurgencies have ended in a variety of different ways. Insurgent and terror groups have been unable to pass the cause on to the next generation; they have lost popular support, transitioned into legitimate political avenues, or been successfully repressed by the established authority, and their leaders have been captured or killed.[43] Many organized crime groups have ended similarly, but they have also been defeated by financial strangulation. No insurgent or terrorist group, however, has been dismantled by rolling up its financial networks. Insurgent and terrorist groups can support their armed struggles in a number of ways. For example, states can sponsor them, as can charities, sympathetic communities, and even other armed groups. But because an organized crime group is a profit-seeking entity at its core, governments that have focused a long-term campaign directed at a cartel's finances have often caused it to disintegrate. "Indeed, every time a criminal cartel has been challenged with the appropriate level of resources, legal tools, and political determination, it has been defeated."[44]

One often overlooked difference between organized criminal syndicates on one hand and terrorists and insurgents on the other is the use of the money. When it comes to financial gain for terrorist and insurgent groups, money is an investment in violence; for organized crime, money is an investment in making more money.[45]

The economics of contemporary terror organizations are, therefore, very similar to those of a state, whereby wealth generated by the nation is distributed to keep the community going. In contrast, a criminal organization operates like a private corporation, the ultimate goal being profit and accumulation. The monetary flows of a criminal enterprise are managed through an accountancy system regulated by balance sheets similar to those of a big corporation. . . . [Terror groups] are more interested in money disbursement than in money laundering; for one, revenues generated by their legitimate businesses do not need to be laundered, they need to be distributed within the network of cells and sleepers.[46]

To be sure, a drug cartel will disburse money to their members and pay for weaponry, security, and personnel proficient in the use of violence, but this is part of the cost of doing business, rather than the business itself. The rise in sophistication of weaponry and expertise among the Mexican cartels is largely because they are in competition with each other and the state over control of illicit narcotics.

The proponents of the narco-insurgency/narco-terrorism school are equating low-intensity conflict with what might be better labeled as "high-intensity crime."[47] John Mueller uses this term to describe criminal acts (like looting, raping, trafficking in illicit goods) that occur during intrastate conflicts that distort the political objectives of some warring groups. However, the term, rather than its meaning, works well to describe the Mexican trafficking organizations and their particular form of extreme gangsterism and violence. Instead of being warring groups that are turning to criminal activities as a means to keep their struggles alive, criminal groups in Mexico are turning to warlike activities to keep themselves in business. Mexico is not suffering from an insurgency or terrorism. The purpose of the violence by cartels in Mexico is quite different. One person's gangster is not another person's terrorist or insurgent.[48] Although insurgent, terrorist, and criminal violence each challenge the authority, legitimacy, and capacity of the state, they do so for differing reasons that should not be conflated. By the actions of challenging the authority of a government, all terrorists and insurgents are criminals, but not all criminals are insurgents or terrorists.

The ongoing violence in Mexico cannot properly be called terrorism or insurgency, but it is more than just a crime wave or a crime spree by a street gang. High-intensity crime involves criminal activities that are more violent and widespread in their scope and that are usually, but not always, sustained over a long period of time. A crime wave is generally a sharp uptick in illegal activities that is geographically isolated to a single city or section within a city; it is also relatively brief and does not necessarily include increases in violence but can include such things as a rash of burglaries and thefts. Mexico by contrast has suffered multiple and sustained outbreaks of violence like murders, extortion, kidnappings, and mutilations perpetrated by at least seven cartels and over two dozen enforcement groups and gangs in several cities over a prolonged period of time.

Beyond Mexico, there have been other cases of high-intensity crime, including Colombia's struggle against the Medellin and Cali cartels from 1980 to the mid-1990s; post-Soviet Russia's battles with the *mafiya* from the early to mid-1990s; and Italy's crackdown on the Sicilian Mafia in the early 1990s. The outbreak of high-intensity crime in these cases reveals similar structural causes with Mexico—a change in the political-criminal nexus, the emergence of new illegal opportunities, and a more confrontational stance by the state. In the case of Colombia, the Medellin cartel tried to expand its reach into Cali's markets as the Colombian government launched a crackdown against the Medellin cartel.[49] Pablo Escobar declared war against the government and attacked a wide array of civilian and state targets. The collapse of the Soviet Union and the Communist Party removed social and political control mechanisms that had allowed elite exploitation of organized crime while keeping the level of violence under control. The traditional *vory-v-zakone* mafia groups were challenged by newer, more entrepreneurial criminals; competition erupted among ethnic criminal groups (particular Slavic groups versus groups from the Caucasus); and competing organizations fought for dominance in particular sectors of the economy. The Sicilian Mafia in the early 1990s attacked the Italian state in retaliation for a betrayal of the long-term exchange relationship with the Christian Democrat Party in which political protection was traded for electoral support. This was manifested in the killings of magistrates and a broader campaign of intimidation, targeting innocent civilians and some of Italy's historic monuments.

A situation of high-intensity crime does not mean that a war cannot occur. But it is a war of a different kind. It is an armed conflict fought by criminal groups over what are essentially criminal goals; the groups are confronted by the state while their goals are rejected by it. In fact, many of the antagonists, including the Mexican president as well as the cartel leaders, have explicitly called the situation a war. Moreover, there are several conflicts occurring at once that blend into each other.

There is the conflict of cartels among each other, the conflict within cartels, cartels against the Mexican state, cartels and gangs against the Mexican people, and gangs versus gangs. When combined, they form a mosaic cartel war that creates an atmosphere that appears to many as "somewhere between Al Capone's Chicago and an outright war."[50] It is not an irregular or regular war; neither is it a small war, nor a general war, nor a limited war, nor a total war, nor any of the familiar appellations given to armed conflicts fought by conventional militaries. And, finally it is not "a war about nothing."[51]

A mosaic cartel war may appear to fit the description offered by proponents of "new wars."

Martin Van Creveld argues that war has become "transformed" as we enter a "new era, not of peaceful competition between trading blocks, but of warfare between ethnic and religious groups" waged "not by armies but by groups whom we today call terrorists, guerrillas, bandits and robbers." Barbara Ehrenreich, too, points to a "new kind of war," one "less disciplined and more spontaneous than the old," and "one often fought by ill-clad bands more resembling gangs than armies." In a similar vein, Mary Kaldor writes about "new wars," ones centrally about "identity politics," fought in a context of globalization by "a disparate range of different types of groups such as paramilitary units, local warlords, criminal gangs, police forces, mercenary groups, and also regular armies including breakaway units of regular armies."[52]

But this is just another description of low-intensity conflict. This merely describes the contemporary ways in which low-intensity conflicts are waged and who fights in them. It is not articulating an alternative environment where a war can still occur.

Because it is a war of a different kind in Mexico, the targets of the cartels have been wide ranging—from police to journalists, from clinics to discos, from military bases to children's birthday parties. "Criminal cleansing" has occurred in Mexican towns where cartels have ordered residents to leave or face possible death. A mosaic cartel war is complex in its manifestation and confounding to traditional military and law enforcement solutions. As a result, there is great difficulty for governments on either side of the border to fight this type of war and to bring the violence under control. As R. T. Naylor argues, "The violence of the state is often a response to the violence of the criminal; the reverse is also true. And once the interactive cycle of violence is set in motion, it may be impossible to separate action from reaction, or to say for sure if the reduction in the use of violence on one side will lead to the same on the other."[53] This frustration over cause and effect is part of the reason that many have used inappropriate labels from other types of conflicts to describe the situation in Mexico. "The nub of the problem, then, is that iron responses to violent nonstate actors of all types and character . . . are no substitute for case-specific, strategic judgments."[54] An alternative conception is required to more accurately describe and assess the current outbreak of a mosaic cartel war in Mexico, its dynamics, and its potential end.

The Violence of High-Intensity Crime: War of All against All

The lumping together of insurgents, terrorists, and organized criminal syndicates under the overly broad category of nonstate actors adds little analytical clarity. Defining a term in opposition to another term—such as nonstate as opposed to state—is conceptually murky. Many disparate groups can be classified as nonstate actors, ranging from multinational corporations to civic organizations. Adding the qualifier of "violent" does little to ease the confusion because violent nonstate actors can include sea-going pirates as well as private military companies. The term "network" is more descriptive than nonstate actor. It refers to the structure and operation of a group, but once again it encompasses a wide variety of groups that are both legal and illegal. The term "dark network" focuses on how nonhierarchical, dispersed social structures are used for criminal ends.[55] Although an improvement, the term describes a structure and a process rather than the actors or the conditions they use collective violence.

Differing groups are organized under certain conditions to use collective violence to achieve a particular goal or set of goals. Table 1.1 details the differences between low-intensity conflict, which the violence in Mexico has so often been confused with, and high-intensity crime. In Mexico, as with the outbreaks in Colombia, Russia, Italy, and Japan, high-intensity crime is due to a war waged by *violent entrepreneurs who seek to prevail over one another and the state in a hyper-competitive illegal market in order to control it or a particular portion of it*. Violent entrepreneurs are mostly private groups that create "a set of organizational solutions and action strategies enabling organized force (or organized violence) to be converted into money or other valuable assets on a permanent basis. . . . Violent entrepreneurship is a means of increasing the private income of the wielders of force through ongoing relations of exchange with other groups that own other resources."[56] For violent entrepreneurs, the use of force is the extension of private profit making, rather than the extension of a political agenda. Violence itself is a means, not an end; it is "a resource, not the final product."[57] Drug cartels are a type

TABLE 1.1

	Low-Intensity Conflict	High-Intensity Crime
Main Actors Challenging the State	Irregular Forces —Guerrillas, Insurgents, Paramilitaries, Militia, Terrorists	Violent Entrepreneurs —Organized Criminal Syndicates, Cartels, Gangs, Vigilante Groups
Primary Motivation of Actors	Politics, Ideology, Religion, Ethnicity	Illicit Profit, Personal Enrichment
Primary Goal of Actors	Territorial Autonomy, Control of Government, Access to Resources, Repel Occupier	Maintenance and/or Expansion of Power in Illicit Economy
Environment of Organized Violence	Political, Ideological, Social, Economic Spheres	Hypercompetitive Illegal Markets
Cessation of Violence	Victory, Reconciliation, Armistice, Peace	Co-optation, Elimination, Management, Break-Even Point

of violent entrepreneurship because they derive their income from the use of force to prevail in private activities that are highly circumscribed or prohibited by the state. As a resource, violence is used by cartels to insure that the product, which is illegal in nature, is delivered to its client base so that profits can be derived.

With their abilities to use the contours of NAFTA to expand their trade in illegal drugs, to manage the decline in the previous patronage relationship with the PRI, to outmaneuver the PAN's direct challenge to their existence, and to streamline cocaine smuggling from the Andes to the United States and beyond, Mexico's cartels are entrepreneurial in the most traditional sense because they have exploited change in order to create new service and business opportunities. They have engaged in what business expert Peter Drucker has called "purposeful innovation" by managing risky ventures in new and systematic ways and by creating novel capacities that generate steady, and in some cases increasing, wealth.[58]

Drug trafficking is a highly risky venture. Due to the product's illegality, it is "vulnerable to lawful seizure as well as to theft; property rights cannot rely on written records and are generally poorly defined; liability is restricted to the physical person; individual mobility is greater; and agents are tougher, more prone to risk, and more secretive than their law-abiding counterparts."[59] When it comes to markets for illegal products, like those for marijuana, heroin, cocaine, and methamphetamine, avenues for conventional legal dispute settlement are not available to participants. When an illegal deal is broken, the parties cannot go to court to seek remedy, nor would any remedy be legally enforceable. The main consequence for those operating in illegal markets is far reaching: because there is no legal arbiter or legitimate enforcer to guarantee an agreement among the participants to produce or deliver the commodity, all transactions related to illegal markets are surrounded with violence or its potential use. In short, those who wield violence most effectively act as the ultimate arbiter in any dispute.

However, most of the time "illegal drug markets are generally peaceable."[60] Violent entrepreneurs involved at the higher end of the trafficking network often behave peacefully and cooperate with one another while colluding with state agents. This is another element that separates violent entrepreneurs from insurgents, guerrillas, and terrorists. Namely, interactions among violent entrepreneurs (and the state in many cases) are characterized by considerable cooperation.[61] While this may belie the term "violent entrepreneurs," it does not detract from the use of force as the means of ultimate arbitration should cooperation break down. This is dramatically demonstrated in a hypercompetitive illegal market, which has a number of characteristics. First, the commodity is not only illegal and its delivery illegal, but the market size for the commodity is great and the number of violent entrepreneurs seeking to control the commodity or its delivery is numerous. Second, there is a lack of a powerful arbiter to enforce agreements among violent entrepreneurs. Third, the state actively engages in curtailing the market and a spin-off criminal market emerges as a result of the competition over the primary commodity in dispute. All of these factors create the conditions for the outbreak of war among violent entrepreneurs who seek to prevail under these conditions, thereby raising the overall levels of violence in society. The situation comes to resemble Hobbes's state of nature, an anarchic condition of a war of all against all.

Narcotics trafficking is the perfect example of a hypercompetitive illegal market because marijuana, heroin, cocaine, and methamphetamine are illegal products, and their delivery to market is illegal. Although this market is often peaceful, it not infrequently becomes highly susceptible to the use of violence by the participants.[62] Disputes can arise over price, purity, delivery times and location, personnel, territory, payment, seizure, theft, and secrecy. With 1,500 metric tons of marijuana, 15 metric tons of heroin, 200 metric tons of cocaine, and 20 metric tons of meth coming from Mexico yearly,[63] the sheer volume of illegal narcotics combined with the number of cartels and gangs creates areas for possible contention and risk at a geometric rate. In addition the stimulation of a consumer market in

Mexico is now a $1 billion market; according to a drug survey conducted by the Mexican health ministry, over 50 percent more Mexicans have become addicted to illegal drugs now—some 465,000—than in 2002.[64] With a high number of violent entrepreneurs operating and competing within and for the same territory, the ability to generate a long-standing balance of power among them is transient. Alliances are ad hoc and made for convenience, but often deteriorate.

The scale of the drug trade, the number of competitors, and shifting alliances (as well as the active interdiction efforts by the United States and Mexico) help explain why the cartels possess such sophisticated weapons arsenals and have advanced tactics. They have been forced to increase their acquisition of higher-end firearms and intelligence-gathering technology to mitigate short-term and long-term risk exposure.[65] Some of the firepower that Mexican authorities face from cartels and gangs is the same that U.S. soldiers encounter in Iraq and Afghanistan, including improvised explosive devices. The introduction of Colombian cocaine was especially pernicious. The long supply chain to get cocaine from the Andes into North America is difficult to guard, exacerbating security issues that require more firepower and intelligence to mitigate.

Closely related to the multiple areas of contention and risk is the second characteristic of a hypercompetitive illegal market: more vicious competition when there is no arbiter powerful enough to impose order (like a corrupt state, a dominant cartel, or a concert of cartels) or when long-standing arrangements among cartels and with state officials have deteriorated (as seen in the case of PRI) or when the state actively seeks to curtail the market through forceful intervention (as with the PAN). In such an environment, "sellers compete, not by improving quality or reducing prices, but by acquiring more efficient violent skills in order to enlarge their share of the market."[66] A former agent with the DEA described how Mexican cartels have behaved as a result of the lack of an arbiter: "They would kill people who didn't cooperate. They would kill people who didn't pay a fee or a toll (for moving drugs through their territory). They would kill people who were not necessarily disloyal to them. They killed them to set an example."[67] The pressure from both the U.S. and Mexican governments has only heightened the atmosphere of uncertainty for cartels. When the agents of the government begin to actively challenge groups operating in the market or seek to drastically reduce the market's power, cartels have an incentive to resort to force for the protection of themselves and their livelihoods.

Cartels in hypercompetitive illegal markets can actually be more violent than terrorist or insurgent groups, meaning that high-intensity crime can result in a greater rate of death and misery than some low-intensity conflicts. Mexico once again reflects this—the level and intensity of cartel violence has been much worse than that of the Zapatista insurgency during its heyday in the mid-1990s. In fact, more people have been killed by Mexican cartels since 2006 than were killed by the Irish Republican Army and Loyalist groups during the decades-long "Troubles" in Northern Ireland (over 3,500) and exceeds the number of deaths inflicted by Turkey's long-running PKK insurgent group (over 12,000). And the city with the world's highest murder rate remains Ciudad Juarez, Mexico.

Finally, hypercompetitive markets are also characterized by other collateral crimes like kidnapping and contract killing that are submarkets spawned by the competition over the illegal commodity in dispute. Enforcer groups such as gangs are often hired to kidnap and kill those who have reneged on a deal or to kidnap and kill the relatives who are related to the participants involved in the initial dispute. Much of the spillover violence in cities like Phoenix, Tucson, and San Diego is the product of this ancillary market. These activities become another source of illicit income and profit with all the consequences, pressures, and points of contention of the main market of illicit narcotics. In Mexico, kidnapping is one of the least punished crimes; it rose 15 percent in 2010 and has tripled since 2006.[68] These ancillary activities, in effect, become another market to fight over. For example, a portion of the violence in Tijuana during 2008 was related to a dispute over the Arellano Félix Organization's expansion into kidnapping.[69] The result of these additional submarkets is the exacerbation of the intensity and scope of violence.

For governments, combating violent entrepreneurs in hypercompetitive illegal markets is different from fighting insurgents and terrorists. There are clients and demand drivers to be considered in battling them that are different from dealing with insurgent or terrorist networks. Counternarcotics, counterinsurgency, and counterterrorism operations are not the same. Merely because they share a common prefix does not mean that they can be employed toward a common end. Notions of victory, defeat, armistice, and peace, which are conditions in low-intensity conflicts, are not necessarily suitable for high-intensity crime. Wars can end, but crime rarely does. And drug trafficking has been especially difficult to eliminate, reduce, or control. In those cases where governments have succeeded in capturing leading drug traffickers and disrupting their networks, they have merely created an opportunity for other criminal enterprises to capture vacated market share.[70] Governments can reduce high-intensity crime by managing the hypercompetitive characteristics of the illegal markets and by eliminating and co-opting violent entrepreneurs in order to mitigate the negative effects on society. An adviser to President Calderón described the government's perspective: "It's like a rat control problem.

The rats are always down in the sewers; you can't really get rid of them. But what you don't want are rats on people's front doors."[71] Governments can also pressure violent entrepreneurs to face a "breakeven point" where cartels begin to view violence as costing them more in profit. Nonetheless, while violence might be reduced, the illegal markets themselves have endured in many cases.

Understanding the Mosaic Cartel War in Mexico

The enduring quality of illegal markets in Mexico requires a deeper understanding of how and why drug trafficking organizations and their associates are fighting with each other and the government. Along with this is the need to examine the effects in the United States and what can be done to address the issue of high-intensity crime next door. While not the same as wars in low-intensity conflicts, cartel wars, in broad strokes, share some common characteristics with all wars—there are organizational structures, leaders, fighters, battlefields, tactics, strategies, and counterstrategies. However, these characteristics take on a different form because of the criminal, rather than political, nature of the struggle, which is multidimensional, multiparty, and occurring in many locations across Mexico. The subsequent chapters continue to address the question about why Mexico has become much more violent as well as addressing the questions of who are the perpetrators of the violence, how and where do they employ it, what are the effects in the United States, what are the current responses, what are some possible outcomes, and what can be done to stem the violence. Forming the spine of this study are the concepts needed to answer these questions about the characteristics and wide-ranging ramifications of the contemporary Mexican cartel wars.

Chapter 2 discusses the strategic reasons that cartels as violent entrepreneurs use physical force in their operating environment. The operating environment of Mexican cartels is not akin to that of al Qaeda, Colombia's FARC, or Spain's ETA. Cartels are not a military either (even taking into account the military background of those in Los Zetas). By delving more deeply into the corporate logic of cartels, Mexico's upsurge in violence can be seen more clearly. With the drug trade concentrated in the hands of seven major cartels and with the barriers to entry so high, this chapter also covers the key players in the drug violence. It discusses the emergence of the Sinaloa, Gulf, Juarez, Tijuana, Beltrán-Leyva Organization, Los Zetas, and La Familia Michoacana/Los Caballeros Templarios cartels, their alliances, and their divisions. While Mexico fits the pattern of other cases of high-intensity crime, it nonetheless possesses unique characteristics. Therefore, the chapter will also examine other societal and cultural drivers of the violence in Mexico.

Chapter 3 expands on the examination in chapter 2 by discussing how the bat-tlefields of the cartel wars are in essence zones of contested authority within hyper-competitive illegal markets. Not all of Mexico has been plunged into drug-fueled violence. Some states and cities are the sites of high rates of homicide while oth-ers are low. To explain the discrepancy, this chapter explores the concept of "geo-criminality." Certain geographical areas facilitate drug operations and hence generate the ability of cartels to satisfy their customer base and thereby earn profit. Without territorial control, a cartel's vulnerability increases, and its ability to sustain itself as an organization is jeopardized. This chapter examines how geo-criminality has turned cities, towns, and neighborhoods into the battlefields of these groups. The chapter also describes how violence is conducted in these areas and some of the targets of the cartels' violence.

Because the "battlefields" in Mexico extend northward across the border, chap-ter 4 explores the increase in crime and the rising numbers of narco-refugees in U.S. cities and towns. Both public safety and public health are being increasingly burdened by cartel activities in the United States and Mexico. U.S. teenagers are being drawn into drug running and gang activities; U.S. law enforcement is show-ing signs of corruption; gang fights are occurring in schools; and national parks are being used to grow marijuana for cartels while shared rivers are now scenes of pirate attacks.

The violence in Mexico and the spillover effects in the United States have not gone unanswered by decision makers in each country. Chapter 5 describes and analyzes the current policies and strategies that are being employed by the United States and Mexico to reduce violence and suppress drug trafficking. Although the Mérida Initiative—a multiyear $1.4 billion dollar program—has been highly touted by both countries as an important milestone in relations between the United States and Mexico, it has not gone unanswered by cartels. The chapter argues that the corporate logic of the cartels is being met by the institutional logic of law enforcement. The clash of these competing logics has increased the uncertainty of all parties and further heightened the violence in Mexico. There is a fragile bal-ance between the dilemmas that policymakers face that, so far, has produced a stalemate at best.

Stalemates have been broken in a number of ways in other outbreaks of high-intensity crime. Chapter 6 looks at a number of possible near and long-term devel-opments in Mexican cartel violence: "the new abnormal"—violence will be an enduring fact in the relations between the United States and Mexico that will require constant management; "the accidental narco"—the Mexican government will pick a side in the cartel fights in order to reduce the violence but will act as a type of enforcer for the cartel; "pax narcotica"—the cartels will make peace among themselves or the strongest cartels will prevail and ask the government to back off in exchange for a reduction in violence; "Zeta state"—the Mexican government will lose legitimacy over time, forcing Mexicans to migrate in greater numbers to the United States or seek out private sources of security in Mexico that can guarantee their safety. The chapter concludes by discussing the warning signs that might signal a "strategic shock" for U.S. and Mexican leaders.

Because the situation in Mexico taking a turn for the worse would have dire consequences for the United States, there is the need for a broader look at solutions to the cartel wars. The Obama administration's *National Security Strategy* clearly makes the case: "Stability and security in Mexico are indispensable to building a strong economic partnership, fighting the illicit drug and arms trade, and promoting sound immigration policy."[72] In May 2010, the president dispatched twelve hundred National Guard members to the border, and in July of the same year, another thousand were deployed for a year as a way to rein in drug trafficking activities and their associated violence. But as Ryan Grim, author of *This Is Your Country on Drugs*, puts it:

> In reality, there is no such thing as drug policy. As currently understood and implemented, drug policy attempts to isolate a phenomenon that can't be taken in isolation. Economic policy is drug policy. Healthcare is drug policy. Foreign policy, too, is drug policy. When approached in isolation, drug policy almost always backfires because it doesn't take into account powerful economic, social, and cultural forces.[73]

Chapter 7 examines the possibilities for comprehensive approaches to remedying drug violence in Mexico. The United States has spent more than $2.5 trillion over the past forty years, yet drug use has remained constant, with ebbs and flows based on shifts in the types of drugs consumed. As long as this demand continues, there is a high likelihood that cartel violence will also ebb and flow unless other, more comprehensive approaches are considered. Such comprehensive approaches should include "high-intensity law enforcement" that serve a larger strategic goal that emphasizes the end of the mosaic cartel war by reducing the hypercompetitive nature of the illegal drug market shared by the United States and Mexico.

At this moment, few dampening pressures exist to bring to cartel wars to a conclusion that is favorable to both the United States and Mexico. In fact, there are more dynamics that will likely lead to an increase in the intensity of violence and its spread farther northward. As an economic resource, drugs have been injected into the sinews of Mexican politics and society, with wide-ranging effects on the overall health of the Mexican state. The health of the Mexican state, with its population of over 100 million, is of acute concern to the United States. If its health declines because criminal violence continues, increases, or spreads, the U.S. government, along with local communities within the United States, will feel an even greater urge to act. As former U.S. attorney Pete Nunez said, "What happens on one side [of the border] quite often affects what happens on the other side."[74] The United States has not been spared from the violence, and as the main consumer market for illicit narcotics, it also bears responsibility for fashioning a response that recognizes not just the spillover effects but the deep-seated American demand for intoxicants. Given the ever-increasing cruelty of the cartels, the question is how to design the best policies that support effective strategies to support justice, human rights, and prosperity on both sides of the border.

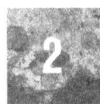

THE "WARRIORS"
Cartels and How They Fight

The uniqueness of Mexico's bout of high-intensity crime is in part the result of the dialectical relationship between Mexico's weak institutions and America's strong demand for illegal drugs. Mexico, like other developing states, suffers from capacity gaps and functional holes, meaning that it fails to provide essential services and maintain an adequate degree of social control. However, the inability of Mexico's developed northern neighbor to stem its own demand for illicit intoxicants has only worsened this condition by supporting a hypercompetitive illegal market that the Mexican government is incapable of eliminating or moderating. Violent entrepreneurs like cartels and gangs have been able to take advantage of the gaps and holes by filling the demand for illegal drugs but in the process have brought with them an extraordinary level of violence and corruption that further diminishes the competence and legitimacy of the Mexican state. Agents of the state, like politicians, attorneys, and police, have been killed or have fled to the United States; members of civil society like journalists and businesspeople have been murdered or kidnapped. The resulting weakness of Mexico's political and legal institutions, along with its compromised civil society, have created a fertile environment of impunity for drug traffickers where there is no inhibition to participating in ever-escalating levels of violence.

The previous chapter covered the broad structural reasons for the outbreak of the contemporary cartel wars—the signing of NAFTA, the end of the PRI's political dominance, the PAN's confrontation of cartels, and changes in the patterns of drug trafficking. A mosaic cartel war that involves gangs versus gangs and cartels fighting against each other, within themselves, against the Mexican state, against street gangs, and against the Mexican people needs to be brought into sharper relief so that the effects on U.S. national security can be better understood and Mexico's gaps and holes can be more properly addressed by policymakers. Like other wars, a mosaic cartel war includes actors who use violence in a particular manner as a way to achieve a particular end. Because this is a multidimensional and multiparty conflict, this chapter seeks to not only answer the question of who perpetrates the violence but also address the questions of why and how they do so.

The leaders of Mexico's cartels are individuals who have less in common with men like Osama Bin Laden or Che Guevara. Rather, cartel leaders have more in common with Al Capone, who was described as a "businessman of crime [with] lucid, rational, and discoverable reasons for his actions."[1] Cartels composed of violent entrepreneurs have an operating environment—the hypercompetitive illegal marketplace—that creates a corporate logic that provides the "lucid, rational, and discoverable reasons" for their particular actions. As violent entrepreneurs, most organized criminal syndicates prefer to operate in the shadows to accumulate profit, unnoticed, ignored, or supported by the state. They also seek to work unhindered by rival competitors and yet must maintain organizational cohesion over time. "To accomplish both their strategic and tactical objectives, cartels must keep police and soldiers at bay, out-terrorize rival cartels, silence reporters and eye-witnesses, keep lawyers from prosecuting and prevent investigators from investigating."[2] To reach these objectives a cartel may resort to violence and, in some cases, war. Some of the violent acts are familiar patterns of war with military-style tactics, targeting, and use of high-powered weapons. The combination of equipment, expertise, and personnel allows cartels to conduct operations that mirror those of professional militaries. Cartels and gangs have set up ambushes for rival cartels and state agents. They have armed convoys to protect the transportation of drugs; they use intelligence and surveillance for security and to plan new attacks. They also conduct information operations aimed at swaying the opinions of rivals, the government, and society.

But other techniques do not resemble "battles." So pervasive is the cruelty of the cartels in Mexico that a unique lexicon in Spanish has emerged to describe some of their acts:

- *Decapitado*: decapitation
- *Descuartizado*: quartering of a body, carving it up
- *Encuelado*: body in truck of car
- *Encobijado*: body wrapped in blanket
- *Entampado*: body in a drum
- *Enteipado*: eyes and mouth of corpse taped shut
- *Pozoleado* (also *Guisado*): body dissolved in acid, looks like Mexican stew.[3]

Choosing various displays of physical force is part of the calculations of corporate logic that are inherent to violent entrepreneurship. In addition, there are other drivers of Mexico's cartel wars that go beyond a group's corporate logic. As R. T. Naylor suggests, society and culture are important influences on violence in illegal markets.[4] These drivers do much in separating high-intensity crime in Mexico from incidences of high-intensity crime in other countries where the body count has been much lower than that perpetrated by Mexican cartels. Also, each of Mexico's seven major cartels employs corporate logic in similar settings, but with differing expressions. Taken together, these factors provide greater detail for understanding the contemporary situation in Mexico.

Five "Laws" of a Cartel's Corporate Logic

As mentioned in the preceding chapter, a cartel is not a military force, neither regular nor irregular. This means that a cartel and its various opponents are not fighting a conventional or unconventional war in Mexico. A cartel is organized to pursue different goals and operate in a different environment than militaries, guerrillas, or terrorists. To succeed in navigating within their operating environment, cartels generally adhere to five "laws" of corporate logic that define their enterprise and help to protect themselves from internal fragmentation, external challenge, and potential elimination.

Law 1: Act to Fill a Demand, but Stimulate Other Markets

A cartel is organized to fill a demand for a difficult-to-acquire product or a difficult-to-provide service that will earn profits greater than those from legitimate sources and through legal means. In effect, the only law that a cartel does not break is the law of supply and demand. As covered in the previous chapter, the demand in the United States for marijuana, cocaine, heroin, and methamphetamine remains both high and illegal, leaving little question about the profitability of a cartel's enterprise. In 2009, the U.S. Department of Health and Human Services estimated that 21.8 million Americans aged 12 or older are illicit drug users; this estimate represents 8.7 percent of the population aged 12 years old or older.[5] The United States is still the leader of the world in the consumption of illicit narcotics. The cartel's goal is to continue to supply this demand, or customer base, and reap the profits. By far, the biggest moneymaker for the cartels is marijuana, which generates an estimated $8.4 billion in annual sales.[6] This is followed by cocaine at $3.9 billion, methamphetamine at $1 billion, and heroin at $400 million.[7] The cartels not only meet the demand for drugs in the United

States, but they also meet the demand of many Mexicans who seek to enter the United States illegally. Before 1995, independent human smugglers, or "coyotes," would arrange for Mexicans to be clandestinely moved into the United States; cartels and gangs would merely "tax" them for using their routes. However, since then, cartels have increasingly moved in to this lucrative territory themselves to the tune of roughly $2 billion a year.[8] They have also combined both narcotics trafficking and human smuggling. Traffickers will often use groups of illegal immigrants to "probe" routes to see if they are safe to use for the smuggling of drugs.[9] Also, traffickers will force those who want to enter the United States to carry drug loads on their person.

Additionally, in a hypercompetitive illegal market where the main source of revenue is up for contention, extortion and kidnapping are ways to earn money for arms, training, and personnel that can be used against rivals and the state. Cartels will hire gangs to engage in extortion, kidnapping, and assassinations of rivals and state agents. Jose Luis Pineyro, an organized crime analyst from Mexico City's Metropolitan Autonomous University, studied the pay rates for hired guns and found that "they're hired for an average of U.S. $500 to $650 a month to kill an unlimited number of people or to carry out other acts of violence. Ten years ago, a hired assassin charged U.S. $12,000 to $13,000 to kill just one person."[10] This price decline reveals that there are not only a large supply of willing recruits and a large number of targets, but that killing someone is cheap option for drug traffickers. Such a low price also contributes to the violence because the expense to a cartel is not an obstacle, and the supply is "disposable and recyclable."

But cartels and gangs will often create their own markets.As violent entrepreneurs who wield coercive force as a resource, they can engage in activities—such as extortion, kidnapping, assassinations—that are not necessarily connected to providing highly sought after commodities to a wanting public. Shaking down businesses for "protection" money, kidnapping businessmen and professionals for ransom, and murder-for-hire schemes can occur without any linkages to the drug trade. These stand-alone, profit-making activities are the equivalent of "a parallel tax system that threatens the government monopoly on raising tax money."[11] The pay received by gangs likely acts as an incentive that perpetuates violence.[12]

Law 2: Use Purposeful, Directed Violence Rather than Random Acts of Violence

To continue to generate profits from illegal acts, an organized criminal syndicate traditionally seeks to operate like a legitimate business by opting for a low profile.

As the famous American gangster Meyer Lansky put it, "Ford salesmen don't shoot Chevy salesmen." In fact, much of the time, organized criminal syndicates choose to avoid violent displays. "The implication is that organized crime violence, while certainly more than an anomaly, is not the norm."[13] Too much violence can be bad for business because it interferes with the group's moneymaking activities and can bring unneeded state intervention. H. Richard Friman argues that "violence serves as a selective tool of market regulation. The selective rather than uniform use of violence reflects in part the potential cost of its use, ranging from retaliation in kind from competitors to greater levels of interference in the market by state authorities."[14] In fact, operating in an illegal market that is unregulated and therefore anarchic often means that a cartel will resort to violence as a way to continue the shroud of secrecy. The desire for secrecy explains why journalists have been targeted in Mexico—reporting the acts of cartels and gangs draws more attention to them.

Thus, the second law of a cartel's corporate logic is the preference for purposeful and directed violence rather than random and capricious violence. As discussed in chapter 1, a cartel uses violence to enforce a deal or as a way to discipline the cartel's workforce of employees, suppliers, and clients.[15] But a cartel also uses force for a number of other strategic and operational reasons. It will use violence for issues of internal security; its members will engage in violence against each other to move up in the organization; and the cartel will resort to force to compete for market share against other cartels.[16] A cartel will also use violence to enhance its reputation. All of these are exacerbated in a hypercompetitive illegal market where paranoia and mistrust over possible detention or death permeate a cartel. In this environment, a cartel is willing to use higher levels of violence by expanding its target list in order to prevail.

Violence is often used for internal security reasons. Because a cartel's activities are subject to detection by law enforcement and challenge by other cartels, loyalty within the organization is highly prized. The presence of an informant, defector, or self-interested member can undermine the ability of the group to make a profit or lead to its possible elimination. It is a "villain's paradox" where a "criminal needs partners who are also criminals, but these are typically untrustworthy people to deal with."[17] Breaking through this paradox often means "breaking bones"; force is a logical option to coerce a possible turncoat into confessing his status or removing him from the organization in a more permanent manner. *Sicarios*, or hitmen, are often from gangs and are employed by the cartels to handle the disloyal. With so many cartels and gangs in competition, along with more confrontational state institutions, Mexico's cartels cannot take internal security as a given and are especially susceptible to concerns about internal security. Mexico's drug traffickers have reason to use force within their own ranks as a purging operation.[18]

Violence used in this manner may also serve as a warning to other members of the group who might also consider defecting. Yet these warnings are not always heeded; disputes over promotion and succession within the group can still lead to killings among its members. If an individual feels frustrated or dissatisfied with the current leadership or the distribution of benefits among the group, there is little to prevent a violent challenge. Lower-level members can use violence for upward mobility.[19] In fact, when a government becomes confrontational by using a "king-pin strategy" of arresting top cartel leaders, violence has often increased because succession issues among the remaining members are open to competition. The larger these "vacancy chains," the greater the uncertainty about succession, roles, and responsibilities within the group and the greater the uncertainty about relationships external to the group.[20] This can lead to splits within the cartel and violence among the members. Further, other cartels may choose to support one faction against the other. All this serves to raise the overall level of violence.

The challenge of maintaining loyalty is at times as important as, and yet also intertwined with, the imperative of competing with other violent entrepreneurs. Preventing traitors is often predicated upon ensuring that money is still flowing to members of the cartel so that they remain satisfied with their participation and stay committed to the group. As such, a cartel must maintain its share of the illegal marketplace, expand it, or move into new areas to do so. Any of these options may prompt a war if a compromise with rivals cannot be arranged. This is partly the case in Mexico, where several cartels were allied with each other in the past before falling out. For example, in 2001 a cartel known as El Milenio was allied with the Sinaloa cartel to control the drug trade in Michoacán. The Gulf cartel in association with Los Zetas invaded in order to secure a larger proportion of methamphetamine market and prevailed over El Milenio. The Beltrán-Leyva Organization also allied with the Gulf cartel and the Zetas against "La Federación" of Sinaloa.[21] Competition over routes, whether to smuggle drugs, people, guns, or money, among various gang affiliates can also lead to violence. The risk of apprehension and loss of a load along one of the smuggling routes into and out of the United States means that other groups using the same route may also be exposed. To protect their routes from interlopers or the incompetent, smuggling groups of all sorts are becoming increasingly better armed.

But pressure from government anticorruption efforts has also exacerbated competition by forcing Mexican cartels to jockey for plazas. Efforts to reduce the number of plazas do not necessarily lead to a consequent reduction of supply or demand; they merely complicate delivery. This complication acts as strategic stimulant for the use of more violence to gain access to a diminishing number of routes. A zero-sum game for a cartel is thus created—it either controls a particular route or it does not. A lack of control reduces a cartel's income, creating the possibility of dissent in its ranks and making the group look weak in the eyes of competitors who may decide to poach territory, assets, or personnel. This is partly the reason that many of the acts of violence have been directed against police and the military in Mexico. Cartels want to prevent them from directly intervening in a cartel or gang battle that might be occurring nearby or to communicate their displeasure at being targeted by security forces whom they believe are favoring rival cartels.

This leads to the final reason a cartel will resort to violence: to enhance its reputation. Violence is often meant to send a message; "a primary goal of communication, namely to modify people's beliefs about a situation or a person, is often better achieved by deeds than by words. Actions send signals and are often meant to."[22] In Mexico, horrific acts like decapitations in discos, displaying heads in soccer fields, and sewing a rival's face to a soccer ball all serve as signals to rivals and to the government.[23] They are a cartel's version of "shock and awe."[24] As Jorge Chabat puts it, "This is psychological warfare. These beheadings serve to stun. They cut them off *to show us what they are capable of.*"[25] The effect is to gain a reputation for ruthlessness that will make a cartel more credible, perhaps forestalling the future need to use violence and to achieve a level of security to continue its operations. It is akin to what Thomas Schelling called "vicious diplomacy."[26] Cartels are often even more explicit in their signaling; dead bodies in Mexico are often displayed with written notes. Known as "corpse messaging," these notes explain who committed the murders and why the victims were killed and include taunts and warnings of future violence.

Law 3: Corrupt State Agents through Incentives or Intimidation
Closely related to the second law of directed violence is the third law of corporate logic: corruption and intimidation of state agents through "*plata o plomo,*" meaning "silver or lead"—silver symbolizing money for a bribe and lead meaning a bullet, symbolizing injury or death. To continue their actions unobstructed by the state, a cartel will corrupt public officials through incentives or punishment. In a cartel war, the state must be co-opted or cowed. This is clearly happening in Mexico. Mexican authorities claim that drug-trafficking gangs pay around 1.27 billion pesos (some $100 million) a month in bribes to municipal police officers nationwide.[27]

In 2010, approximately 3,200 Mexican federal police officers, almost a tenth of the force, were fired under new rules designed to weed out corrupt cops. On the other hand, those who are not corruptible are threatened or executed; a total of 915 municipal police, 698 state police, and 463 federal agents have been killed.[28] Cartels not only operate outside the law; they seek to bring the law into the service of their interests. In an example of silver and lead being used together, a retired army general who was hired to assist the city of Cancun to deal with drug gangs was tortured (his wrists and ankles broken) and then killed. The main suspect was the Cancun police chief, who was paid off by a cartel.[29]

Law 4: Develop and Employ Soft Power

Maintaining group cohesion and drawing recruits is also a required function of cartels. Much like combatants in other types of wars, cartel and gang members will kill to protect the group and kill in its name. But because a cartel is not a military force or an insurgent group, no ideology binds it together, making command and control a difficult issue. While the threat of violence or its actual use can keep a group together, a cartel will also have and wield substantial "soft power" that appeals to members of the organization and to outsiders who may desire to join it. A compelling set of reasons must be provided for an individual to endure a life filled with the possibility of incarceration, bodily injury, and death. As Italian-American organized crime leader Joe Bonanno said, "Mafia is a process not a thing." This reflects the fourth law: there must be the nurturing of a group dynamic for successful organized criminal activities not only to be successful, but indeed to be organized. Trust among the members is integral, and "long-term relationships between illegal entrepreneurs as well as stable criminal partnerships prove to be easier to establish and to maintain among people already bound by blood ties, by membership to a brotherhood, or by common ethnic, religious, or political background."[30] In Mexico, trust and bonding among the members within the Tijuana, Juarez, Sinaloa, Beltrán-Leyva, and Gulf cartels has been generated by family ties, while many other members are from the same city or state. Los Zetas, on the other hand, bond because they share a previous military experience, and La Familia has created its own version of robust born-again Christianity to indoctrinate its members. Prison also fills this function. Many gang and low-level cartel members met in prison, where trust was built over time and where their "credentials" and bona fides were established.[31]

Amid the poverty in Mexico, the ability to earn a living as well as the opportunity to be viewed as a person of status are powerful enough incentives to join and stay in a cartel or gang. As one resident of Reynosa put it:

They're [killing] for kudos. They're doing it to show that they can wear this T-shirt by this designer worth this much money. It's like stripes on a military uniform. You walk around and everyone knows what rank you are, because your T-shirt is worth $300. It's a system of rank: if you have this T-shirt, you get a cute girl to show off; if you have an even more expensive T-shirt, you get an even cuter girl. But you can't be seen in the T-shirt you wore last year, which has gone out of style—that would mean you hadn't climbed the ladder. Same with the mobile phone and the SUV—you have to have the latest.[32]

Cartels and gangs are able to take advantage of the poverty in Mexico to recruit members and maintain some degree of group cohesion. Participating in a gang or a cartel as a hired killer is not only a means of earning money; it also permits a degree of professional mobility that is rarely found in the few occupations in Mexico. Mexican hit men are in the business because they hope to climb the criminal ladder and eventually become cartel leaders themselves. "Being a paid assassin has proven to be the best criminal profession from which to attract the attention of drug bosses and start a trafficker career."[33] The Mexican attorney general Arturo Chavez-Chavez summed up the social conditions and the consequent ability of cartels to use them for soft power purposes:

The dynamic engine of crime in our country is not the issue of ideology; it is not that [cartels and gangs] are seeking to amend the structures of the political system. In Juarez, what is happening is that we are measuring the consequences of social breakdown that began long ago in that city. In these criminal groups, many of their members stress the fact that they only identify with the organizations to which they belong; they do not identify with the nation much less the region. But they have a strong group identity with the gang to which they belong, and consequently, the rules and law they respect are those which this group operates.[34]

From insignia on vehicles used in attacks on rivals and police to tattoos that reveal their loyalties, cartel and gang members are able to demonstrate a sense of belonging. Videos on YouTube are also made to celebrate the laudable acts of the group, further building a sense of community within the organizations.

Law 5: Cultivate Community Support or Acquiescence

A cartel needs to maintain a relationship with the community at large so that citizens at least permit or do not actively obstruct criminal activities. Cultivating community support or at least acquiescence is the fifth "law" of crime group's corporate logic. A cartel can be predatory with certain members of the community, but only to a certain degree. Many organized crime groups will build links within the community in order to gain support and to shield its members from harm. Criminal groups "build schools, health care clinics, lending services at decent rates; they pay for funerals of widows—all of this gives them legitimacy. So people begin to 'protect' criminals. . . . People buy into the community that gives these kind of protective structures."[35] Some cartels in Mexico are able to demonstrate their benevolence by throwing festivals, donating items to the poor, and standing up for residents who have been wronged by the government authorities in the past. On the other hand, a cartel will also use hard power to instill fear in a community to gain acquiescence and freedom of action. Witnesses to crimes are threatened, and attacks against innocent bystanders are used to intimidate citizens into accepting the presence of a cartel in a particular area. Cartels in Mexico use *narcomantas* to communicate directly with society. Narcomantas are banners displayed in public places with messages for the community, rivals, and the government. The messages often report news of cartel activities and atrocities by rivals as well as contain taunts or threats.

Beyond Corporate Logic: Other Drivers of Mexico's Mosaic Cartel War

Not all the violence that is gripping Mexico can be explained by corporate logic; the positing of rational actors using cost-benefit analysis who decide what actions will best achieve a desired end for their organization is only one facet that explains the scope and magnitude of the mosaic cartel war. Violent entrepreneurs, as human beings, are subject to a wide range of impulses and pressures that drive them to aggressive acts of viciousness. In Mexico, there are a number of societal and cultural elements that make some drivers of the violence unique. These macro-level drivers add an important contextual layer upon the corporate logic of the cartels' actions.

Narco-Cultura

There is a strong countercultural tide in Mexico. *Narco-cultura* makes drug trafficking and its associated crimes appear acceptable and even admirable. For many young people in Mexico, it is cool to be a drug trafficker. There is the phenomenon of "narco jr.," or college kids and "townies" who know the exploits of dead smugglers and gangsters while seeking to emulate their style.[36] *Narco-corridos* are music ballads that celebrate the exploits of cartel members; the music videos on

YouTube and Facebook also extol their virtues. These bands are linked to particular cartels and gangs; members will often commission a song in commemoration of a fallen comrade to be played at his funeral.[37] So meaningful are *narco-corridistas* to the cartels that they are often targeted by rivals; over ten were killed between 2007 and 2010.[38] These are attacks on the morale of a rival cartel. Narco-culture also includes the co-optation of religious symbolism through narco-saints, which give members spiritual legitimacy and support for their activities. Jesús Malverde is often referred to as "the patron saint of drug traffickers"; he is an amalgam of a folk hero and Mexican cinema star of the 1940s. Traffickers will pray to him as they do their activities. His likeness is often carried by smugglers, gang members, and cartel members as a way to protect them from danger. So pervasive is his likeness among traffickers that possessing a Malverde icon was ruled by a U.S. appellate court as a legal basis for probable cause that can be used by law enforcement.[39] Another very popular figure is Santa Muerte, or Holy Death, who is a mixture of Catholic symbolism with the pre-Hispanic entities of Mictlantecuhtli and Mictlancihuatl, Lord and Lady of the Dead.[40] Among many prisoners, tattoos of Santa Muerte are popular.[41] Many cartel and gang members commit their acts as offerings to Santa Muerte in exchange for a good death when their time comes.

The Cycle of Revenge and Machismo Competition

Revenge is also a motivation for members of cartels in Mexico. Much of the violence is intensely personal in nature and is not necessarily an outgrowth of the profit motive. Attacks between cartels are often about settling scores and grudges. This sort of violence is more akin to blood feuds over honor. Machismo and family ties combined with violence often have led to a cycle of vengeance and reprisals that has proven difficult to stop.

Machismo is also connected to the apparent competition of one-upmanship among cartel members and their gang enforcers. Each grisly murder on display may also be viewed as an attempt to outdo the previous exhibition. Mexico's current cartel war "is fought through YouTube and mobile phones as well as backroom torture chambers. Cartels and killers use YouTube to threaten rivals and public officials, and boast of their killings, or set up rogue websites to broadcast their savagery. . . . Images of murders, mutilations, and executions are posted on the Internet as a blend of sado-pornography, prowess, and sick humor."[42] These are duels combined with spectacle. "It's a social performance, a performance of power, of very male power."[43] This "male power" is bound up in a macro-level driver of violence: in Mexico there are high numbers of young men, many of whom are unemployed or underemployed. Mexico is the eleventh most populous country, with over 100 million people; nearly 50 percent are males under 25 years old, which is also the median age,[44] but males under 25 have the highest rate of unemployment.[45] These men are prime recruits for cartels and gangs as well as the main perpetrators. As Peter Reuter puts it, "Violence is a young man's game" because they are the ones who generally engage in violence more than do their older counterparts.[46]

"Machisma" on the Rise

The violence in Mexico is not the exclusive domain of men; in fact, incarceration rates for females have increased yearly. Women fill a number of other roles in cartel wars. They act as spies who gain intelligence from law enforcement and rival cartel members by using seduction. Women are often used as diplomats to parlay deals with state agents and other cartels, and are authorized to kill their counterpart if negotiations fail.[47] Women have proven to be just as ruthless as their male counterparts and in some cases were more so in order for them to prove themselves to male superiors and subordinates as being worthy of their positions.[48] There are also women who have risen to high levels of certain cartels and have perpetuated, rather than lowered, the violence. These "queenpins" such as Sandra Ávila Beltrán, known as La Reina del Pacifico (Queen of the Pacific), Edith Lopez-Lopez or La Reina del Sur (Queen of the South), Ivonne Soto Vega or La Pantera (the Panther), and others rose to prominence because of several factors related to the corporate logic of a cartel. First, vacancy chains created by government intervention removed senior and mid-level male leaders from cartels and paved the way for competent women to step in and run certain aspects of cartel operations. Second, the importance of family and trust were key enablers for the participation of women leaders. This guaranteed a certain level of cohesion and certainty that men who were not related to each other by blood could not provide. Third, law enforcement officials were not conditioned to think of women as cartel leaders but as victims who were pawns of their male relatives or husbands. This allowed some cartel activities to escape detection, thereby enhancing operational security.

Street-Level Experience and Professional Expertise

Vacancy chains not only lead to disputes within cartels over succession, but they have also meant that more violent lower-level foot soldiers and their lieutenants have moved up in the organizations. These men earned their "stripes" on the street, where solving disputes through violence is common. This makes them more likely to choose violence as an option in any confrontation. The Mexican Ministry of

Defense (Sedena) claims that one out of three traffickers has a military background and that former police also form a large proportion of cartel membership.[49] Choosing violence as an early option is a hallmark of Los Zetas, who are proficient in the use of violence as a matter of their previous professional expertise. This infusion of former security personnel has raised the levels of violence. One of the most pernicious elements introduced to the hypercompetitive illegal market was the use of active-duty and former police officers as enforcers by the Tijuana cartel. To counter this move, other cartels raised the stakes; the Juarez cartel created its own enforcers, La Linea, while the Gulf cartel employed former members of the Mexican military, Los Zetas, as its armed wing. Although the cartels were violent before Los Zetas began their association with the Gulf cartel, the use of military-style tactics, operations, and strategies created a type of innovator's dilemma for the other cartels. They either had to mimic Los Zetas or be at their mercy. Even Los Zetas felt the pressure of their own successes and recruited Guatemalan special forces, Kaibiles, into their ranks in order to fend off the other enforcer groups.

Proximity to Supplies of Arms
A type of arms race has gripped the drug trade in Mexico. Since 2006, Mexican authorities have confiscated over 86,000 weapons from cartels and gangs.[50] Not only are there many former security professionals who comprise sizable portions of the cartels, but they also have access to a number of venues where they can acquire high-end weapons. Guns and ammunition are purchased at American gun shows. "Straw purchasers" of American citizens who have clean criminal records that can pass background checks are paid by Mexican gang members to buy guns on their behalf. These weapons are routinely used by the cartels to kill soldiers, police officers, competitors, and traitors. Of the 29,284 firearms recovered in Mexico in 2009 and 2010 and submitted to the Bureau of Alcohol, Tobacco, Firearms, and Explosives (ATF) National Tracing Center, 20,504 were from the United States.[51] The ATF claims that the vast majority of the traced weapons come from the four U.S. states along the border, with Texas first, followed by California, Arizona, and New Mexico.[52] This is due to the more than 6,600 licensed dealers that operate along the border.[53] However, many military-style weapons come from the arsenals that remain from the civil wars in Central America. Rocket-propelled grenades, mines, and high-caliber guns are imported from countries such as Guatemala and El Salvador. Security personnel who have deserted also bring arms with them when joining a cartel or gang. These weapons in the hands of the untrained pose a threat, but when placed in the hands of the highly trained, who can operate as an integrated unit, violence then becomes much deadlier.[54]

Getting "High" on Their Own Supply

In Mexico, there are reports that many low-level cartel and gang members are intoxicated on drugs; they use the drugs that they traffic. This helps to explain the gruesome nature of many killings; they are easier to commit while intoxicated. "They're disgusting people, high on amphetamines."[55] Videos on YouTube and Facebook show members taking drugs and celebrating their recent actions against rivals and police. The gruesome murders "occur while they are consuming their product. They are not sober. They are operating in a group, they are drugged up, and they are operating with a sense of absolute impunity."[56] The lack of restraint in some of the killings is the product of intoxication and can lead to a type of "carnival" atmosphere where enforcers are encouraged to get high as a reward for their work.

Mexico's Major Cartels

Corporate logic and other macro-level explanations of violence provide the framework for understanding how and why high-intensity crime in Mexico has reached proportions that create an atmosphere of war. The following section provides the various distinctions among the cartels and serves to highlight some of the most notable examples of how each cartel acts in accordance with the corporate logic of a violent entrepreneur in a hypercompetitive illegal market. The origins of the cartels and their primary motivations for using violence reveal their essential criminal nature while showing how their acts still constitute a form of warfare. Although there are other smaller cartels, seven groups and their gang affiliates are responsible for the bulk of the killings in Mexico: Tijuana, Gulf, Sinaloa, Beltrán-Leyva Organization, Juarez, Los Zetas, and La FamiliaMichoacana/Los Caballeros Templarios.[57] Each of the cartels is unique in character and has taken various positions against rivals and the state; some are older, and some originated as offshoots from other cartels. Their strategies, operations, and tactics have shifted over the years for various reasons related to corporate logic and other factors that are unique to Mexico. As the war goes on, and depending on which of the cartels survive, their actions will likely take new forms but still conform to the patterns associated with being violent entrepreneurs seeking to prevail in a hypercompetitive illegal market.

Tijuana Cartel (Also Known as the Arellano Félix Organization)
Founders: Ramón Arellano Félix, Benjamín Arellano Félix, Francisco Rafael Arellano Félix, Carlos Arellano Félix, Luis Fernando Arellano Félix, Eduardo Arellano Félix, Francisco Javier Arellano Félix

Gang affiliates: Fuerzas Especiales del Muletas (FEM), Sicarios, La Eme, Logan Calle 30, 18th Street, Varrio Chula Vista, Sur-13, Wonderboys, Border Brothers

The Tijuana cartel is an example of violence created by a vacancy chain, internal struggle over succession, shifting alliances, machismo, the role of women, and a cycle of revenge. The Tijuana cartel was an exceptionally violent cartel before 2006 but is now one of the least powerful of the cartels. The cartel was implicated in the 1993 assassination of Catholic cardinal Posada Ocampo as well as the killing of DEA agent Enrique Camarena in 1989. It is also known as the cartel that employed "El Pozolero," or "the soupmaker," who earned his named by reportedly dissolving three hundred bodies of the cartel's victims in acid. While trafficking mostly in marijuana, it also traffics cocaine, heroin, and methamphetamine and has diversified its criminal activities to include human smuggling, murder for hire, kidnappings, and auto theft. It is also an example of how a cartel will gravitate back to the second law of corporate logic by reducing its use of violence once a threat to its profit-making is lessened.

The split in the Tijuana cartel in the 1980s between Miguel Angel Félix Gallardo (the "godfather") and Hector Palma has led to nearly twenty years of nasty fighting because Palma aligned with Chapo Guzman of the Sinaloa cartel. In 2008, Guzman was still focusing on the Tijuana cartel by aligning with a faction of the cartel after the arrest of the only Arellano brother not dead or imprisoned.[58] In 2008, Tijuana was beset by extreme violence. At its height, one hundred executions occurred in one week. This was largely the product of a vacancy chain created by the arrests of the all the Arellano Félix brothers. Without the bonding of close-knit family ties, the remaining members engaged in a vicious fight over who would control the plazas in the state of Baja California. One faction reached out to the Sinaloa cartel. Known as the Garcia faction, they were considered by law enforcement to be a proxy of the Sinaloa cartel.[59] A narco-corrido included the verse, "We'll show you what real war is like."[60] Much of the violence in Tijuana can be blamed over this factional fighting. However, there was also a personal and machismo dimension to the violence. After the killing of the girlfriend of the Garcia faction's leader, a killing spree against the opposing faction and members of Los Zetas was launched as a reprisal.[61] Not to be outdone by men, two of the sisters of the original Arellano Félix family have played prominent roles. One sister is the mother of Luis Fernando Sánchez Arellano, the leader of the faction who stood against the defector. The other manages the finances of this same faction.[62]

The violence began to subside after the arrest of the leader of the Garcia faction, Teodoro Garcia Simental, in January 2010. The number of homicides in Tijuana dropped, partially as the result of the arrest, which has allowed the other faction to engage in "mopping up" operations that do not require large displays of violence. There is a lower level of violence because the dominant faction is using 9mm handguns instead of large automatic weapons and kills its opponents on the outskirts of the city in order not to draw attention to their activities.[63]

Gulf Cartel

Founders: Juan Nepomuceno Guerra, Juan García Abrego, Arturo Guzmán Decena, Jesús Enrique Rejón Águila, Jaime González Durán, Heriberto Lazcano, Miguel Treviño Morales

Gang affiliates: Grupo Tarasco, Los Numeros, Texas Syndicate, Mexikameni, Hermanos Pistoleros Latinos (HPL), Tango Blast

The Gulf cartel is an example of shifting alliances, competitors seeking to expand their market share, corruption and killing of state agents, the cultivation of community support, and vacancy chain infighting. It is also responsible for raising the levels of violence in Mexico to previously unknown heights when the cartel's leader in the late 1990s brought in former members of the Mexican special forces to act as bodyguards and assassins. Known as Los Zetas because of the its leader's designated radio call sign of "Z1," they used violent tactics previously unheard of in Mexico's narcotics industry: the group launched rocket-propelled grenades in the streets, murdered police officials, and attacked employees at the city's largest daily newspaper because they were unhappy with the coverage.[64] The recruitment of Los Zetas demonstrates the importance of protecting cartel interests from rivals' challenges and from state efforts to interdict smuggling loads and to shut down the cartel. It also demonstrates the desire of the Gulf cartel to expand its influence into areas controlled by other cartels.

A substantial amount of the Gulf cartel's power stemmed from Los Zetas, which allowed the Gulf cartel to control a vast amount of territory to move marijuana, cocaine, heroin, and methamphetamine to different markets in the United States unhindered by competitors or law enforcement. This team of former military men "led the charge in the 2004 to 2007 battle between the Gulf and Sinaloa cartels for control of the Nuevo Laredo corridor, one of the most profitable smuggling access points into Texas."[65] In 2003, there was a short-lived alliance between the Gulf cartel and a portion of the Tijuana cartel that was negotiated in prison. Two years later, the alliance dissolved due to a personal dispute between leaders, and the Zetas were dispatched to Baja California to eliminate the Tijuana cartel.[66] Although one of the Gulf cartel's leaders, Cardenas Guillen, was arrested in 2003, he was still able to run a sizable portion of illegal operations from jail by bribing and extorting prison authorities. He continued to cultivate community support by throwing "Children's Day" festivals in a number of cities that included clowns, wrestlers, desserts, and toys.[67]

The Gulf cartel also uses plata o plomo in combination with narcomantas against state institutions. For example, in late 2008, state prosecutors in Michoacán found a head in an ice chest with a message, "From the Gulf Cartel," and two weeks later, as a follow-up, six funeral wreaths were displayed in the streets of Hermosillo with hand-lettered posters that read: "This is a message for the entire state police force, if you mess with us we are going to kill you and your entire family."[68]

Cardenas Guillen's extradition to the United States in 2007 prevented him from continuing his leadership role and led to a succession battle among the more violent second-tier cartel members who earned their reputations as enforcers. The rather light sentence that was given to Cardenas Guillen in February 2010 "suggested that Cardenas sang, gave names, details," which heightened the uncertainty within the alliance between the Gulf cartel and the Zetas and among their respective members.[69] Los Zetas, who were initially involved in the succession battles by supporting certain factions against others, quickly broke away from their former employers to chart an independent course that included the seizure of vast amounts of Gulf cartel territory. The Gulf cartel formally announced the dissolution by hanging narcomantas in Matamoros that read, "The Gulf Cartel distances itself from the Z[etas]. In our ranks we do not want kidnappers, terrorists, bankrobbers, rapists, child-killers, and traitors."[70] But the relentless pressure from the Zetas and the Sinaloa cartel diminished much of the Gulf cartel's power by mid-2010.

Sinaloa (Also Known as the Pacific Cartel or the Guzman-Loera Cartel)
Founders: Héctor Luis Palma Salazar, Joaquín Guzmán Loera, Adrián Gómez González
Gang affiliates: Los Numeros, Los Pelones, La Gente Nueva, Los Lobos, Fuerzas Especiales de Arturo, Mexicles, Artista Asesinos

The Sinaloa cartel is an example of one of the early beneficiaries of the opening of trade due to NAFTA and the shift in Colombia, cocaine smuggling. For over twenty years, the Sinaloa cartel participated called itself a "Federation" of a number of small drug-trafficking organizations. In 2008, it split into rival factions, including the Beltrán-Leyva Organization. The Sinaloa cartel also demonstrates how sharp increases in violence can be attributed to the zeal to win in a hypercompetitive illegal market by choosing a strategy of dominance. The cartel is responsible for a large portion of the high-intensity crime that Mexico is experiencing because of its desire to act as the main arbiter of a large portion of the illegal narcotics market. Led by the elusive Joaquin "El Chapo" Guzman, the cartel sought to expand its influence at the expense of other cartels who controlled plazas into the United States. It is responsible for a number of gruesome killings that have sought to serve as warnings as part of this campaign; the cartel is responsible for stitching the face of a Juarez cartel member to a football with the threat to eliminate the entire Juarez cartel: "Happy New Year, this will be your last." As head of Mexico's largest cartel, Guzman was also listed as one of the world's top billionaires by *Forbes* magazine.

Much of the violence in Ciudad Juarez is caused by this ongoing battle for dominance of the plazas in the city. But there is also a personal grudge held by El Chapo due to the jailhouse killing of his younger brother allegedly ordered by the Juarez cartel.[71] The Sinaloa cartel also continues to attack Los Zetas in revenge for the killing of El Chapo's prison girlfriend in 2008.

Using the method of plata o plomo, El Chapo was quickly released after his arrest in 1991 when he bribed a police chief with $50,000 in hard cash. His subsequent capture in 2001 was short-lived when he and several other criminals escaped from prison when their electronic cell doors opened without explanation. El Chapo is also active in his community where the cartel routinely employs poppy farmers but also invests in towns with the construction of infrastructure projects.

There are also allegations that the Mexican military is siding with the Sinaloa cartel in its battle against the Juarez cartel.[72] It is unclear whether this is a deliberate strategy by the military or whether they have become subject to plata o plomo overtures by the Sinaloa cartel.[73] By mid-2010, there were indications that Sinaloa had prevailed against the Juarez cartel, but violence continued because of succession issues, the desire for revenge, and continuing government pressure on the cartel. In addition, many shoot-outs are among gang affiliates who are fighting over the remaining areas of profit and are struggling to survive against the onslaught of the new gang infiltrators linked to the Sinaloa cartel.

In the escalation of efforts to control the flow of information and to counter the ability of Los Zetas to wage information warfare, the Sinaloa cartel was implicated in the kidnapping of several well-known national TV reporters in Mexico. The cartel's intent was to force the reporters' station to air videos that implicated police in siding with Los Zetas.[74]

Beltrán-Leyva Organization

Founders: Arturo Beltrán Leyva, Alfredo Beltrán Leyva, Mario Alberto Beltrán Leyva, Carlos Beltrán Leyva, Héctor Beltrán Leyva, Edgar Valdez Villarreal

Gang affiliates: Los Negros

The Beltrán-Leyva Organization (BLO) is an example of a cartel that split from an alliance with another cartel in order to take advantage of more lucrative opportunities. The offshoot group was composed of family members as a way to guarantee loyalty and internal security. However, the BLO has been very susceptible to internal splits due to pressure from the Mexican government and conniving rivals. Vacancy chains have led to the fight for control of the cartel, thereby increasing violence in central and southwestern Mexico. BLO most recently splintered after its leader, Arturo Beltrán Leyva, was killed in a gun battle with Mexican marines in December 2009.

As previously mentioned, the BLO was part of the Sinaloa Federation where it was placed in charge of transporting drugs, bribing officials, and laundering money for the Federation at the time. It also allegedly commanded two groups of hitmen.[75] But in January 2008, Alfredo Beltrán Leyva was arrested by the Mexican army. The speculation was that Sinaloa leader El Chapo Guzman tipped off the government, leading to the killing of El Chapo's son in May 2008 by the BLO. By this time, the BLO had already established its own extensive connections to move Colombian cocaine without the need to include the rest of the Sinaloa Federation. The BLO was able to form an alliance with Los Zetas in order to move cocaine from Guatemala into Mexico and then into the United States.

The BLO is reputed to have one of the best intelligence capabilities of the cartels, with sources placed in high positions within the Mexican government. This was evident when the group killed the family of the Mexican marine who shot and killed Auturo Beltrán Leyva. However, the ramifications of his death continue to plague the group with internal fragmentation. The decision to elevate Hector Beltrán Leyva as the cartel's leader angered Edgar Valdez Villarreal, to whom a sizable portion of the cartel was loyal. The faction loyal to Hector has renamed itself "Cartel Pacifico Sur," or "South Pacific Cartel."[76] This faction also used gruesome killings and narcomantas in its war against Villarreal; four decapitated bodies hung over a bridge in Cuernavaca in August 2010 with a message that threatened: "This is what will happen to all those who support the traitor Edgar Valdez Villarreal."[77] In August 2010, Villarreal was apprehended by Mexican authorities and extradited to the United States to face drug trafficking charges. This led to the collapse of his faction's enforcer group, Los Negros.

Juarez (Also Known as the Vincent Carrillo Fuentes Organization)
Founders: Ernesto Fonseca Carrillo, Rafael Aguilar Guajardo, Amado Carrillo Fuentes, Pablo Acosta Villarreal

Gang affiliates: Los Linces, La Linea, Barrio Azteca, Surenos, Syndicato de Nuevo Mexico, Mexican Clique Killers

The acts of the Juarez cartel demonstrate how violent entrepreneurs will raise the level of violence in an effort to stave off a critical loss or potential elimination. The Juarez cartel has been the source of some of the most high-profile attacks in Mexico's outbreak of a mosaic cartel war. It has taken the most confrontational stance against the Mexican and U.S. governments by violently striking out against law enforcement and the state as a way to dissuade the Mexican government, whom it believes is actively supporting rival cartels. The Juarez cartel used the first car bomb in Mexico's history. Its gang affiliate, Barrio Azteca, is also believed to be responsible for the killing of three U.S. consular employees in 2010, two of whom were Americans. The Juarez cartel is also infamous for running the "House of Death," a site used for the torture and killing of suspected traitors, rival cartel members, and those suspected of helping authorities keep tabs on the cartel. It has also entered other illegal markets to earn revenue to make up for lost income from drug trafficking and to finance its operations against the Sinaloa cartel and Los Zetas.[78]

In 2001, after El Chapo Guzman escaped from prison, many Juarez cartel members defected to Guzman's Sinaloa Federation. However, the personal nature of the violence between the Sinaloa and Juarez cartels can be traced back to 2004, when Vicente Carillo Fuentes's brother was killed allegedly by order of El Chapo, which precipitated the killing of El Chapo's younger brother in prison. The challenge from both the Sinaloa cartel and Los Zetas has made it difficult for the Juarez to maintain control of the plazas. To continue to earn money, the Juarez cartel has branched primarily into kidnapping for ransom, human trafficking, prostitution, extortion, and retail sales of drugs in domestic Mexican markets. Los Aztecas have attacked drug rehabilitation centers and clinics; the victims were from groups working with the rival Sinaloa cartel.[79]

In the first half of 2010, it appeared that the Juarez cartel may have lost the battle against the Sinaloa cartel, but it continues to strike against Mexican security forces that it believes are siding with its rival. Graffiti on a wall of a shopping mall contained a claim of responsibility for the car bomb used against Mexican law enforcement; it read in Spanish: "What happened on the 16 [street] is going to keep happening to all the authorities that continue to support Chapo [Guzman], sincerely, the Juarez Cartel. We still have car bombs [expletive] ha ha."[80] Another message was aimed at the FBI and DEA and was posted in an elementary school in Juarez: "FBI and DEA, start investigating authorities that support the Sinaloa

Cartel. If you do not, we will get those federal officers with car bombs. If corrupt federal officers are not arrested within 15 days, we will put 100 kilograms of C-4 in a car."[81] Two months after the warning, the cartel's enforcer group, La Linea, unsuccessfully attempted to detonate a car bomb with only sixteen kilograms of explosives.

La Familia Michoacana (Split into Los Caballeros Templarios in 2011)

Founders: Nazario Moreno González, Carlos Rosales Mendoza, José de Jesús Méndez Vargas, Julio César Godoy Toscano, Enrique Plancarte, Arnoldo Rueda Medina, Servando Gómez Martínez, Dionicio Loya Plancarte, Rafael Cedeño Hernández, Alberto Espinoza Barron

La Familia Michoacana (LFM) was added to the "kingpin list" of major drug trafficking organizations in 2009 by the Obama administration. After the death of its leader and founder, Nazario Moreno, most of the group disbanded, but several members reformed the cartel under the name Los Cabelleros Templarios (LCT) in March 2011. This offshoot of LFM announced its formation with several narco-mantas placed around the state of Michoacán:

To the society of Michoacán we inform you that from today we will be working here on the altruistic activities that were previously performed by the Familia Michoacana. We will be at the service of Michoacán society to attend to any situation which threatens the safety of the Michoacanos.

Our commitment to society will be: to safeguard order; avoid robberies, kidnappings, extortion; and to shield the state from possible rival intrusions. Sincerely, The Knights Templar.[82]

Along with the banners, LCT made its presence known by hanging two bodies from a freeway overpass in Morelia, Michoacán. By selecting the name Los Caballeros Templarios, which translates as "The Knights Templar," the cartel is trying to continue the narrative of the Christian self-defense of their realm that is represented, in their case, as the state of Michoacán. Their acts and operations still cover the same areas as LFM, and with the help of LFM's sworn enemies, Los Zetas, they have frequently confronted each other in violent clashes in rural areas of Michoacán.

LFM is thought to have its origins in a split from a criminal organization known as La Empresa to capitalize on the growing retail drug market in Michoacán and to take advantage of the plaza's location within 186 miles of half the Mexican population.[83] However, its actual origins are murky, but it became well known in 2006 as the group that began mass beheadings. Unlike other cartels, it is an example of a group that seeks to more actively co-opt the state and civil society through a muscular form of evangelical Christianity. By using religion, it generated not only internal cohesion among its members but a type of soft power that appealed more broadly to other aspects of society, making LFM appear as something other than a criminal enterprise. But the cartel's hard power is equally imbued with a degree of religiosity. In many respects, each murder is not only a message but a sermon. Its version of plata o plomo was unique; the combination of intimidation and acts of goodwill proved effective in earning community support when LFM battled rival cartels and the government. It also used its members, rather than relying on gang affiliates, to distribute narcotics in U.S. retail markets. As such, it had a more direct presence in the United States than other cartels.

LFM had billed itself as a protector of traditional values and says that it seeks to rid its home turf of criminality. The inaugural announcement of its intent came in an infamous incident in 2006 when cartel members tossed five decapitated heads onto the dance floor of a nightclub. The accompanying message read: "The Family doesn't kill for money. It doesn't kill women. It doesn't kill innocent people, only those who deserve to die. Know that this is divine justice." LFM ran a very active propaganda campaign aimed at scaring rivals, gaining the acquiescence of the community, and thwarting government action. All were designed to continue LFM's ability to generate profits from trafficking cocaine, marijuana, and methamphetamine, along with kidnapping, extortion, armed robbery, and counterfeiting.

LFM—and its successor, LCT—is a cartel that comes closest to possessing a type of ideology. As one observer put it, LFM is "a faith-based right-wing populist socialist movement emanating from and orchestrated by an organization that just happens to be a well-armed, well-financed violent criminal enterprise."[84] LCT continues this pattern. Group cohesion and successful recruitment was largely based on the charismatic leadership of Nazario Moreno who, before his death in late 2010, distributed his own version of the Bible to members of the group and to the community at large. Members of LCT remain committed to this practice. Like LFM, LCT requires its members to be drug-free, and its members know the punishment for rule infractions, including execution at the hands of the person who recruited them into the gang.[85] Also like LFM, LCT also provides important community services that the government fails to furnish, such as building schools and drug rehab centers and offering consumer loans. As a result, many members of local communities come to respect cartel and gang members because they have "nice trucks, nice houses, pretty girls, money, power. People fear them. Everybody wants what they have."[86] In fact, when the death of the group's founder was announced, spontaneous demonstrations of grief were reported in Michoacán. A banner of support for his supposed successor was also found hanging in the center of Morelia that proclaimed, "Señor Chango Méndez, Give the federal government hell, but please don't involve civilians, and don't burn cars; they have nothing to do with any of this."[87] With the death of its founder and leader, LFM put out a statement to President Calderón that read in part, "Beware, Felipe Calderón, pray to your holy saint because we come with the blessing of our God. Our God Nazario, may God rest his soul. This will not stop until Familia Michoacana dies. We will never die."[88] By referring to its deceased leader, Nazario, as a god, LFM attempted to create its own unique narcosaint in order to preserve its internal cohesion and soft power.

Like the other cartels, LFM also availed itself of the expertise of security professionals by hiring former members of Mexican and Guatemalan special forces to conduct a three- to six-month training camp for its enforcers.[89] LFM's challenge to the state usually began with a large number of well-armed men arriving swiftly by trucks at a municipal government building. With the local police outmatched, members of LFM would tell the mayor that they "want to work here. There will be no trouble, no crime, no drunkenness, nothing," and then the mayor is paid for his hospitality.[90] But a number of police, state attorneys, and mayors voluntarily joined the LFM because of the order that they brought to an area. This did not prevent LFM from directly attacking agents of the state in retaliation for interfering with the operations of the group. When police detained an LFM member with close ties to its leader, the cartel killed twelve off-duty police officers and stacked their bodies along the side of the road.[91]

Although it espoused itself to be a type of vigilante group that protected local citizens against the evils of the drug trade, LFM acted to secure itself in ways that are similar to the other cartels. For example, it formed alliances with other cartels. At its inception, LFM worked with the Gulf cartel and its enforcer group at the time, Los Zetas. This alliance broke down in 2009, and the LFM began to work with the Sinaloa and Tijuana cartels. Without a firm footing in the northern Mexican states, LFM worked with these cartels mainly as a way to access their plazas for the transport of LFM's drug shipments. However, after Los Zetas declared their independence from the Gulf cartel, LFM rejoined the alliance with the Gulf cartel with the addition of the Sinaloa cartel. LCT appears to have broken this alliance by gaining aid from Los Zetas to mop up remaining elements of LFM.

Los Zetas

Founders: Arturo Guzmán Decena, Jesús Enrique Rejón Águila, Jaime González Durán, Heriberto Lazcano

Gang affiliates: MS-13, MS-18

Operational divisions: Los Halcones, Los Zetitas, El Viejos, Cobras, Los Zetas Nuevas, Las Ventanas, Los Manosos, La Direccion, Las Panteras

Los Zetas were, at their inception, a way for the Gulf cartel to ameliorate many of the negative implications of adhering to corporate logic in a hypercompetitive illegal market. When they were part of the Gulf cartel, Los Zetas "collected debts, secured new drug trafficking routes at the expense of other cartels, discouraged defections from other parts of the cartel organization, and tracked down particularly 'worrisome' rival cartel and gang leaders all over Mexico and Central America."[92] Los Zetas were recruited from the Grupo Aeromovil de Fuerzas Especiales of the elite Mexican counterinsurgency forces by the Gulf cartel. Their insertion into the hypercompetitive illegal market had dramatic effects.

The Zetas were the first Mexican drug trafficking organization to employ a military-grade arsenal, making the jump from the standard AK-47 to shoulder-fired missiles, armor-piercing ammunition, fragmentation grenades, heavy machine guns, and even improvised explosive devices. Some of these weapons are stolen from the Mexican military or purchased on the black market. Most are bought legally in the United States and smuggled across the border. Arguably more important, the Zetas were the first to combine this massive firepower with expertise in infantry squad tactics, complex assaults, and other military techniques. The result has been a qualitative escalation in the intensity of drug-related violence in Mexico.[93]

They very rapidly became one of the "most technologically advanced, sophisticated, and violent of the paramilitary enforcement groups."[94] After their split from the Gulf cartel, Los Zetas continued to structure themselves like a military force, by dividing themselves into operational divisions and relying less on gang affiliates for enforcement work.

Los Zetas also combine this military prowess with techniques aimed at the government and society, making them unlike other cartels. With their military background, Los Zetas are skilled at using information warfare. They pioneered the use of narcomantas that are aimed at drawing more members of the Mexican military into their ranks. One narcomanta that was hung by a freeway overpass in Nuevo Laredo read: "We offer a good salary, food and medical care for your family. Do not suffer mistreatment and hunger. We will not feed you [cup-o-noodles]."[95]

Los Zetas also are quite adept at targeting journalists in order to suppress media coverage. The goal of attacking the media is to reduce the coverage to make Mexican civil society less aware of the activities of Los Zetas and therefore less likely to be able to form opinions and act against the group.[96] In 2011, they expanded their war against information to social media. In that year, Los Zetas committed a cluster of killings of online bloggers who reported on their acts. In Nuevo Laredo, a man who helped moderate a website that posted news of shoot-outs and other Zetas cartel activities was killed and left mutilated at an intersection. A corpse message was left saying that "this happened to me for not understanding that I shouldn't report on the social networks."[97] A female blogger known as Laredo Girl was decapitated in late September 2011, and the brutalized bodies of a man and woman were hung from an overpass earlier that month with a sign saying they had been killed for their online activity. Los Zetas also had a brief feud with the hacking network known as Anonymous. Los Zetas had kidnapped one of the network's members. In retaliation, the group of hackers threatened to expose the personal information of Los Zetas and their associates in government. Los Zetas eventually released the member of Anonymous it was holding with a warning to the network not to test them again.

Due to their reliance on professional military expertise, Los Zetas jealously guard their group identity. Those who pose as Zetas are frequently brutalized as examples to other copycats. In addition, when members of Los Zetas are detained or imprisoned, the group has organized prison raids to free them. The most spectacular raid occurred in 2008, when fifty Zetas dressed as police infiltrated a prison in Veracruz to release five of their comrades. The group identity of Los Zetas is also reflected in narco-cultura through narco-corridos and the worshiping of narco-saints. The narco-corridos in their honor reflect their martial spirit: "We are 20 the group of Los Zetas/united as a family/We are 20 the force/with diplomas of suicide/Aware that in each action/we can lose our life . . ."[98] Los Zetas also honor their fallen comrades by retrieving them from graveyards, making offerings to Santa Muerte, and praying to its likeness for an honorable death.[99]

Because of their military origins and given their start as enforcers, Los Zetas cultivate community support through their mystique as a type of soldiers of fortune. Due to their widespread notoriety for acts of brutality, Los Zetas have a "criminal brand" that is used by other gangs who call themselves Zetas as a way "to exert control over their opponents by sparking fear in them."[100] Their acts are designed to convince people in an area that local politicians, local police, federal authorities, and other cartels are weak and that the real power lies in the hands of Los Zetas.[101]

Los Zetas have also used plata o plomo to this end by getting local police officers to kidnap rivals and deliver them to the organization so that they can be tortured and killed. They routinely mark their victims with the letter *z*, often by carving it into their flesh, as part of their campaign of intimidation. Their start as enforcers has also colored their ways of coping with the pressure put on them by rivals and the state. In order to compensate for the loss of personnel, they have sought to coerce illegal migrants to become smugglers and hitmen. In fact, Los Zetas are responsible for the largest massacre in the cartel wars so far: the killings of seventy-two illegal immigrants in August 2010. According to the lone survivor, members of Los Zetas kidnapped them, robbed them, and gave them the ultimatum to become hired members of the cartel or face death. When the migrants refused, they were gunned down.[102]

They seek to expand their ranks with special forces from Mexico but also increase their proficiency and influence around the region through the recruitment of Kaibiles, Guatemalan special forces. Although now operating as a separate drug trafficking cartel, Los Zetas still contract themselves for hire as enforcers for other cartels and have expanded into kidnapping, money laundering, and arms trafficking.

Warfare of the Cartels

As violent entrepreneurs waging war in a hypercompetitive illegal market by following the corporate logic of their enterprise, the cartels in Mexico have acted in ways that resemble warfare. As seen in the descriptions of the major cartels and their activities, each has organized alliances, employed violent strategies, and conducted information campaigns in order to reach its goals. Although these goals are largely criminal in nature, this has not detracted from the cartels' desire to coerce rivals, the state, and society through the use of deadly force and propaganda. All of these actions conform to the corporate logic of violent entrepreneurs while reflecting the unique characteristics of Mexican culture and history. Mexico's major cartels have demonstrated a number of motivations, such as personal grudges, machismo, and religious expressions of devotion as part of the mix of their actions, resulting in cycles of revenge, one-upmanship competitions, and lurid killings. The result is that the use of violence by the cartels has been less constrained than many other groups like terrorists, insurgents, and guerrillas.

Like other groups engaged in conflict, Mexico's major cartels have formed alliances. The seven major cartels have fractured and reconfigured and continue to be in a high state of flux; this is especially evident with LFM and LCT.[103]

Some alliance formations have reflected balance of power efforts, with cartels seeking to protect their interests by associating with each other against rivals. Alliances were sought after internal divisions within a cartel brought about by arrests or deaths and the subsequent fights over vacancy chains. Alliances were also constructed when one group sought to dominate a certain portion of a market or to control certain key plazas. Balances of power have also been initiated when one group sought dominance, as in the case of the Sinaloa cartel. But there have also been bandwagoning activities where cartels have sought to ally with a powerful cartel, rather than join smaller cartels as a balance, to destroy a rival. By early 2010, there was the brief emergence of the "New Federation," an alliance among the Gulf and Sinaloa cartels along with LFM to destroy Los Zetas. Following the pattern of cartel propaganda, the announcement of the New Federation was made to the Mexican people via YouTube, saying, "Without the 'Z' you will live without fear. . . . If you are a Zeta, run because the MONSTER is coming. . . . The new alliance have raised their weapons to fuck the Zetas because they have undermined the drug trafficking business with their kidnappings, extortions, etc. To sum it up, they don't give a shit about the freedom and tranquility of the Mexican people."[104] As witnessed by the formation of the New Federation, LFM was not beyond engaging in balancing activities, regardless of its espousal of upholding religious values and seeming disdain for drug traffickers. While potentially a "supercartel," this alliance was tenuous at best due to the deep-seated rivalry between the Gulf and Sinaloa cartels. On the other side, the alliance between the BLO and Los Zetas was placed in jeopardy with the capture of BLO leader Edgar Valdez Villarreal by the Mexican military. This may have been a sign that Los Zetas turned on their partnership in a bid to capture all the plazas, but it opened another front for Los Zetas and the potential for infighting within the BLO.

Closely related to the balancing actions of the cartels is the arms race that continues among them. The insertion of the Mexican military into cartel rivalries, along with the introduction of Los Zetas, ratcheted up the competition to outgun the other participants in order to survive. The search for weapons and expertise has been fruitful given a region that is awash in weapons and security personnel. Tactics and operational sophistication have improved over time as each party has increased its armaments and skills. Three new enforcer groups—Cártel de Jalisco Nueva Generación, La Resistencia, and La Mano con Ojos—emerged in 2011 to take advantage of shifting alliances and openings of new territories. One of the newest tactics is the *narcobloqueo*, a road block constructed by gangs and cartels comprised of stolen or carjacked vehicles to prevent the police and military from intervening in gunfights within a particular neighborhood. This has led to the development of fully armored "narco-tanks" with gun turrets and inch-thick steel designed to punch through road blocks and military checkpoints.[105]

Like alliance building and arms races, the application of force by the cartels demonstrates a variety of strategic approaches such as brute force, denial, deterrence, and punishment. When it comes to taking on rivals, brute force has been the most chosen strategy to capture or recapture plazas or to seize drug loads or money shipments. Denial was used in actions designed to prevent the encroachment of rivals by targeting certain members, seizing weapons caches, stealing drug loads and money shipments, and preventing access in and out of plazas. The grisly deaths and mutilations have been used as both deterrence and punishment of traitors as well as rivals. Attacks against the state by the cartels also reflect varying strategies. Small-scale attacks, like the killings of individual mayors or police officers, were brute force operations to remove them from positions of authority where they could obstruct operations. However, they were also punishment in the form of revenge for the arrest of an associate or a group of associates and served as deterrents to honest officials who may have challenged cartel activities. Large-scale attacks, designed to kill as many state agents as possible, were ways to coerce the state to stop it from intervening in the hypercompetitive market by siding with a rival. The grisly nature of many homicides has been used to serve as a deterrent to internal traitors as well as to rivals and state agents who may seek to challenge a cartel.

The attacks against members of civil society reflect the same strategies as those employed against the agents of the state. Kidnappings for ransom and extorting businesses and professionals are brute force ways to earn money; many carjackings are to procure vehicles to use in narcobloqueos. Cartels have also killed individual citizens as punishment for challenging a cartel, witnessing a crime, or being related to a person who has done either. Punishment has also been used against narcocorridistas who are viewed as mere extensions of some cartels and gangs. Large-scale attacks against ordinary citizens have been part of a larger campaign to increase the pressure on the government to ease its stance or to cease its apparent support for a competitor. However, in the case of LFM's grenade attack on Mexico's independence day, an attack against a large number of citizens may have been a way to distract the state and focus its attention on a rival. The targeting of reporters and editors is once again a way for the cartels to hide their activities or coerce the media to report on the misdeeds of a rival. The cartels seek to control information and will intimidate reporters who, out of fear or caution, will write what the traffickers want them to write. This campaign of coercion appears to be working. In September 2010, the editors of the major newspaper in Ciudad Juarez offered a truce with the drug cartels:

To the organizations that are disputing the plaza of Ciudad Juarez: the loss of two reporters of this publishing house in less than two years represents an irreparable breakdown for all of us who work here and, in particular, for their families. We would like it to be known, we are communicators, not psychics. With that in mind, as information correspondents, we want you to explain, What is it you want from us? What is it you want us to publish, or stop publishing? Explain so we can attend to these issues.

You are, at present, the de facto authorities of this city. . . . This is not a surrender. Nor does it mean we will give up on the work we have been developing. This is a respite, an offering of truce to those who have imposed their law on this city, providing they respect the lives of those of us who dedicate ourselves to informing the public.[106]

Violence directed toward the media also may have a deterrent effect; as a form of self-censorship, journalists may simply refrain from publishing the entire circumstances of a particular event.

Cartels have also proved adept at information operations. Through the use of narcomantas, graffiti, videos, and the Internet, the cartels have aimed to shape the way that rivals, the community, and the state view their exploits. Cartel propaganda has contained incentives aimed at potential recruits, but it has also contained threats. Some videos are displays of bravado or help to support the strategies of violence detailed previously. Showing executions or confessions of citizens, rivals, and state agents on video serve to back up deterrent warnings, further campaigns of coercion, and demonstrate the willingness of the cartels to mete out punishment. Tribute videos have been made to eulogize members who have been killed, but they also serve to promote the "soft power" of the cartel by showing the close-knit nature of the group. By attacking members of the media, they have sought to shape the understanding of events in ways that are favorable to their specific group or to reduce coverage, allowing them to work more clandestinely.

These displays of corporate logic by the cartels are not the only ways that the situation in Mexico constitutes a war. Like other conflicts, the regions and territories where the combatants fight are important considerations. The control of territory is also a basic goal of the cartels; this too provides further evidence of the war that is gripping Mexico. Yet the criminal core of the conflict along with its complicated, mosaic nature means that the plazas are not the only areas of contention. Knowing the "battlefields" of the Mexican cartels is the focus of the next chapter.

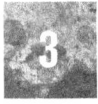

THE "BATTLEFIELDS"
Geography of Violence and Trafficking

The corporate logic of cartels as violent entrepreneurs along with the unique macro-level drivers of Mexican culture and history are also linked to the geography of Mexico, the United States, and the North American region as important factors in explaining the high-intensity crime that is gripping Mexico. This complex combination of factors has meant that the U.S.-Mexico border is a blurry, rather than a bright defining, line that separates two sides. The blurriness has created a rich ecology for criminality. Mexico has a history of supplying Americans' long-standing appetite for illicit substances, from *tequileros* who smuggled liquor into the United States during Prohibition to today's gangs who take narcotics along familiar routes of the past.

Lawlessness south of the United States–Mexico border is nothing new. A culture of crime and banditry has long existed throughout the northern Mexican states and the southwestern United States and has benefited from geographical homogeneity, terrain favorable to criminal activities, impoverished communities easily attracted to enrichment through nefarious means, and a folklore mentality that celebrates the exploits of larger-than-life characters existing outside the law.[1]

In a hypercompetitive market where narcotics are the main commodity in contention, access to territory where it is produced and transported is a key issue in dispute. Drug crops that are used to make heroin and marijuana must be grown, harvested, transported to labs for processing, moved to distribution points, sold to wholesale markets, and purchased at the retail, or street, level. Methamphetamine must be produced with the necessary precursor chemicals and moved along the distribution chain in a similar manner as indigenously grown drug crops. Colombian cocaine and heroin must be received from South America and moved to market. Profit taking is done at each stage of the enterprise, meaning that money laundering is an additional feature of the mosaic war in Mexico. Moving drugs, money, guns, and personnel requires autonomy of action that is only enabled by unfettered access to certain areas—staging points, transit routes, and market destinations. The battlefields of the cartel wars are in essence zones of contested authority among cartels, gangs, and the government within a hypercompetitive illegal market.

These zones are the products of the larger regional context of drug trafficking. Mexico is a hybrid node in the drug trafficking chain that stretches from South America to the United States and Canada, from the Andes to the Arctic. Mexico functions as a transit, source, and demand country. This hybrid quality is unique in the patterns of drug trafficking; this uniqueness is an additional reason that the violence in Mexico has been so intense and has occurred in various cities and towns. The hybrid function of Mexico provides another reason for the mosaic quality of the cartel war—there are more reasons to fight because there is more territory that is important to the production, distribution, and consumption of drugs.

Cartels are fighting over a number of different issues related to this hybrid quality. As a transit country, Mexico suffers from a "location curse" because it lies between cocaine suppliers in South America and the U.S. market. "After being shipped in bulk from Colombia, cocaine is broken down into smaller loads and moved to the northern border where it is re-aggregated into larger shipments."[2] This part of the distribution chain—shipment and smuggling—is where the highest profits are made; nearly a quarter of the price of a kilo is kept as profit. As previously mentioned, border cities such as Nuevo Laredo, Juarez, and Tijuana have a strategic location where the reaggregation occurs and consequently have witnessed intense fighting. Cocaine, in particular, has a far longer supply chain than marijuana and methamphetamine; because the supply chain is transnational, it is difficult to guard. The result, in addition to profitability, is that protection of shipments has made the Mexican cartels involved in the cocaine trade more aggressive and violent than smaller groups that traffic in marijuana or Mexican heroin.[3] As part of the location curse, Mexico is also a source country for marijuana, methamphetamine, and heroin. Cartels and gangs have fought over warehousing issues as well as over production areas. Finally, Mexico is now a consumer market for drugs; one study conducted by the Mexican government found that drug consumption in the Mexican state of Sonora, a key border state for smuggling, had increased by 30 percent in six years.[4] Supply, in some instances, has driven demand. This growth in the Mexican consumer market has created turf-level disputes over street-level sales and control over local retail markets.

While the previous chapter covered the operating environment of the cartels and the corporate logic that it generates, this chapter examines the physical environment where cartels apply their corporate logic and employ strategies of brute force, denial, deterrence, and punishment. Cartels as violent entrepreneurs in hypercompetitive illegal market are fighting over the infrastructure and resources that generate profit. The areas that are essential to the drug trafficking enterprise are numerous, furthering this war's mosaic qualities. The various targets that are attacked by cartels within these areas raise crime in Mexico to the level of high intensity.

The "Geo-Criminality" of Mexico's Mosaic Cartel War

Not all of Mexico is gripped by drug-fueled violence; some areas are bloodier than others. This can be understood as a function of "geo-criminality." While the concept of geopolitics in international relations is "the relation of international political power to the geographical setting,"[5] geo-criminality is the relationship of criminal power to geographical setting. Violent entrepreneurs treat territory differently than actors engaged in low-intensity conflict. For cartels, territory is not about "winning hearts and minds" but access to markets and retrieval of profit. Certain geographical areas facilitate drug operations and hence generate the ability of cartels to satisfy their customer base and thereby earn profit. Without a degree of territorial control, a cartel's vulnerability increases and its ability to sustain itself as an organization is jeopardized. Unlike combatants in conventional wars or insurgencies, violent entrepreneurs in high-intensity crime are not attempting to control territory for political reasons. Their goal "is cash, not sovereignty."[6] Therefore, their perspective on geography is different from groups engaged in armed conflict to gain political objectives; rather, it is based on an economic understanding of power as an outgrowth of illicit profit.

The primary factor in whether a cartel will seek to control an area is its strategic importance to the movement or production of drugs.[7] "Areas of cartel concentration are the area along the U.S. border; coastal port cities on the Pacific Ocean, Gulf of Mexico, and Caribbean Sea; and cities and towns located on federal highways between these points."[8] Map 1 provides a representation of the major cartels' areas of influence, operation, and contention.

Geo-criminality of the Mexican cartels is formed by the heartland, rimland, and periphery that contain Mexican states that are the essential parts of the drug

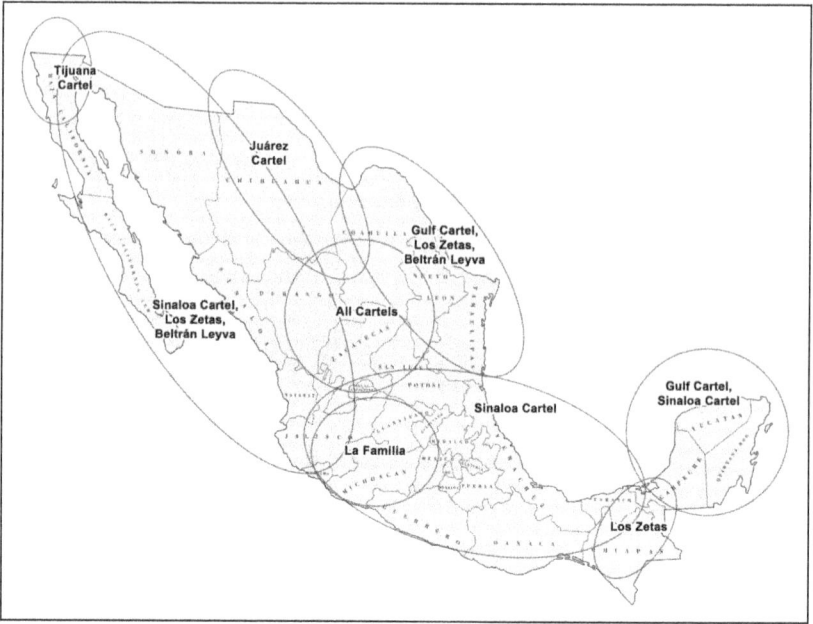

MAP 1   Courtesy of the U.S. Army War College; used with permission.

trafficking network. The heartland, or core, of criminal power for Mexican drug cartels emanates from the states with the lucrative plazas. The heartland is supported by the rimland and, to a lesser extent, the periphery. The rimland is formed by states that contain key drug crop areas as well as areas where narcotics and precursor chemicals are received and transported; the periphery is comprised of states where there are small local retail markets for drugs, refuges for top cartel leaders, and some drug production. The heartland and the rimland form a tight relationship in the movement of drugs, and in some cases, there is an overlap between states in the heartland and rimland when it comes to the cultivation of drug crops or production of drugs. The rimland also serves to supply retail markets in the periphery. The seven major cartels would be able to continue the bulk of their activities without the periphery but would find it exceptionally difficult to do so without the heartland or rimland. Relinquishing or shifting local retail markets or moving the safe havens of the top leadership in the periphery would be easier to do than losing critical nodes in the heartland and rimland. Due to the nature of the supply and production chain of illicit narcotics, the delineations of heartland, rimland, and periphery are relatively unchanging. Control of them, however, is not.

The five laws of the corporate logic of cartels are practiced in varied ways in the different regions to exert control and hence generate profit and power. The use of purposeful, directed violence rather than random acts of violence are most acute in heartland and rimland states. This is largely because cartels are fending off challenges from one another and the government as well as dealing with internal security by guarding against possible splits. Government success against one cartel becomes a business opportunity for a remaining faction or for another cartel, who struggles over the control of a route or territory. State agents have also been targeted through bribery and intimidation in these areas. However, state agents in the periphery have been more subject to bribery than violence. In the periphery, where there are retail markets, the street stakes are lower and the need to maintain zones of refuge has meant uneasy truces among the major players in Mexico's mosaic cartel war. Soft power is expressed throughout Mexico with the ability of citizens to hear narcocorridos or view laudatory videos. Community support is easily cultivated in those areas where the cartels originated; cartel leaders and gang members are often viewed as hometown heroes. The acquiescence of the community is also garnered in areas where cartels and gangs are "headquartered" for trafficking operations.

The Heartland

The heartland is comprised of six Mexican states that border the United States and contain the lucrative plazas: Baja California, Sonora, Chihuahua, Coahuila, Nuevo Leon, and Tamaulipas (see map 2). As previously discussed, with plazas located in these states, the competition among the cartels for ownership and access has been acute. Each of the seven main cartels cannot afford to be locked out of some sort of presence in the heartland. Alliance building and strategies of brute force, denial, deterrence, and punishment have been used by the cartels to ensure freedom of action in the heartland. It is no surprise that four of the major cartels originated in heartland states. Two of the major cartels are named after the cities in the heartland states where they originated—the Tijuana cartel in Baja California and the Juarez cartel in Chihuahua. The other heartland cartel, the Gulf cartel, began in the city of Matamoros, Tamaulipas. Los Zetas were introduced in the heartland due to their association with the Gulf cartel.

The Tijuana cartel is in control of Baja California and has been able to fend off challenges from the Sinaloa cartel that were encouraged by a split in the Tijuana cartel. It has fought mainly a defensive war against the Sinaloa cartel as well as a war to consolidate itself; it has not sought to expand into other heartland territories or into the rimland. The Gulf cartel territory includes Tamaulipas and portions of

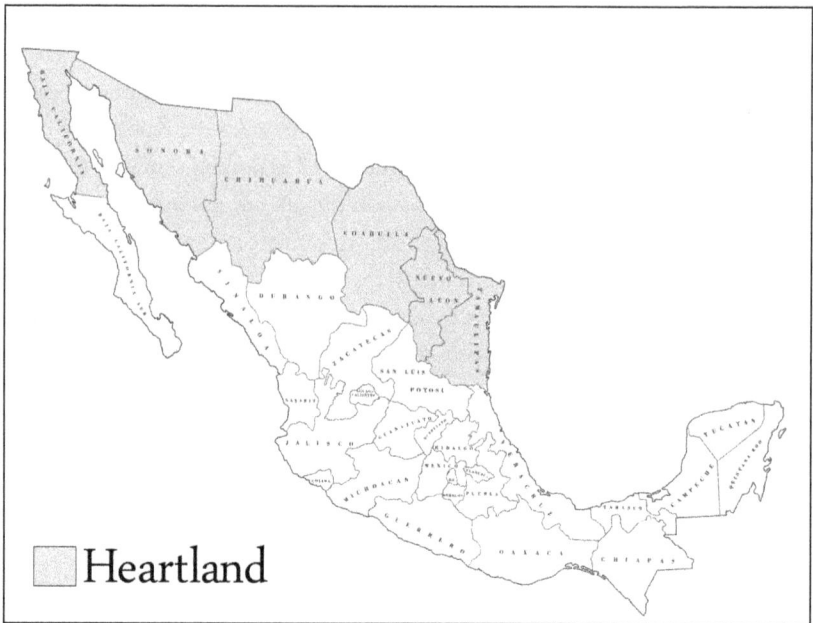

MAP 2   Courtesy of the U.S. Army War College; used with permission.

Nuevo Leon. The Gulf cartel also controls a rimland state of Veracruz where the ports of Veracruz and Tampico are located. Due to their former association with the Gulf cartel, Los Zetas have a widespread presence in the heartland and are under assault by the New Federation to "cleanse" them from this region.

Several cities have been the sites of large numbers of violent deaths. Most notable has been Ciudad Juarez, which has been the intersection of the ambitions of several cartels and their enforcers. Juarez has been the murder capital of the world with an average of nearly 200 homicides per 100,000 residents.[9] It has been the site of some seemingly random acts of violence. Two dozen heavily armed gunmen burst into a drug rehabilitation clinic and killed nineteen addicts, ranging in age from 18 to 25. Suspected cartel hitmen killed thirteen high school students and two adults at a party in Ciudad Juarez.[10] The attack on the clinic was aimed at gang members associated from rival cartels who were seeking treatment, and the attack on the party was thought to be due to mistaken identity. Juarez and El Paso, Texas, represent a primary crossing point for drugs. The Sinaloa cartel's desire to expand its operations has meant the need to seize the drug routes in the state of Chihuahua, which lies to the south of New Mexico and west Texas. Not only has Ciudad Juarez been a prized target, but smaller farming towns through the Juarez Valley that were under the control of the Juarez cartel have also been targeted by the Sinaloa cartel.[11]

Juarez has long suffered cartel violence, but the city of Reynosa, Tamaulipas, is an example of how quickly a city in a heartland state can become a site of intercartel rivalry. In early 2010, over fifty people were killed in a six-week period in Reynosa. Before 2010, Reynosa was a largely peaceful city because top leaders of the Gulf cartel and Los Zetas developed a loose power-sharing agreement in northern Tamaulipas, where Reynosa is located. But the split between the Gulf cartel and Los Zetas made the city a site of contention between the two cartels. The cycle of revenge began in January 2010 when a member of Los Zetas was killed by the Gulf cartel in the city, and the cartel refused to hand over his killer to Los Zetas.[12] Adding to the strife, the Gulf cartel has been joined by its allies in the New Federation to make this city and a good portion of Tamaulipas a focus of their efforts to eradicate Los Zetas. A banner hung in Reynosa's main plaza in early March 2010 addressed to Calderón asked for the withdrawal of the military so that the sides could fight it out among themselves. It was signed by the "fusion of Mexican cartels united against the 'Z' [Zetas]."[13] The overall goal of the violence is to dominate the smuggling routes through northern Tamaulipas and the Rio Grande Valley, from the city of Matamoros in the east to the city of Nuevo Laredo in the west. Reynosa lies between these two cities, and when combined with the city of Monterrey to the south, which moves drugs northward, a broad triangle is formed.

As a result of Reynosa's location, traveling along the triangle is often dangerous. The U.S. Department of State issued a travel advisory urging U.S. citizens to avoid unnecessary travel on Mexican Highway 2 between Reynosa and Nuevo Laredo. Clashes have occurred between soldiers and gang members and cartel enforcers along another highway that connects Monterrey and Reynosa. Not only do drugs, guns, money, and personnel flow along these routes, but the Mexican military also uses them to travel to crime scenes. At times, gangs and enforcers have simultaneously blocked military posts in Reynosa and Matamoros to prevent army patrols from intervening in gang-related shootouts. Human trafficking also occurs along these routes. Within this triangle is where Los Zetas massacred seventy-two migrants from other countries who were transiting through Mexico on their way to the United States.

The Rimland

The rimland is formed by a second group of states that contain key drug cultivation and production areas as well as transit points for narcotics and precursor chemicals: Durango, Sinaloa, Nayarit, Guerrero, Oaxaca, Jalisco, Colima, Aguas Calientes,

Veracruz, Tabasco, Michoacán, Yucatan, Chiapas, Quintana Roo, and Campeche (see map 3). From the rimland, drugs are sent to the heartland in preparation for smuggling into the United States. Most of the rimland, along with a few heartland and periphery states, cultivates, produces, or transits drugs:

- Marijuana cultivation: Michoacán, Chihuahua (heartland), Sinaloa, Durango, and Jalisco
- Poppy production: Guerrero, Sinaloa, Durango, Chihuahua, and Nayarit
- Methamphetamine production: Baja California (heartland), México, Jalisco, Sonora (heartland), Tamaulipas (heartland), Michoacán, Nayarit, Sinaloa, and Durango

South American cocaine and heroin come overland through the states along the southern border shared with Guatemala, but the bulk of Andean cocaine and heroin is shipped by air or boat along two main routes. The first route enters the Yucatan Peninsula via remote airstrips or the port of Cancun, and the second route enters Mexico via port cities in Guerrero and Michoacán.[14]

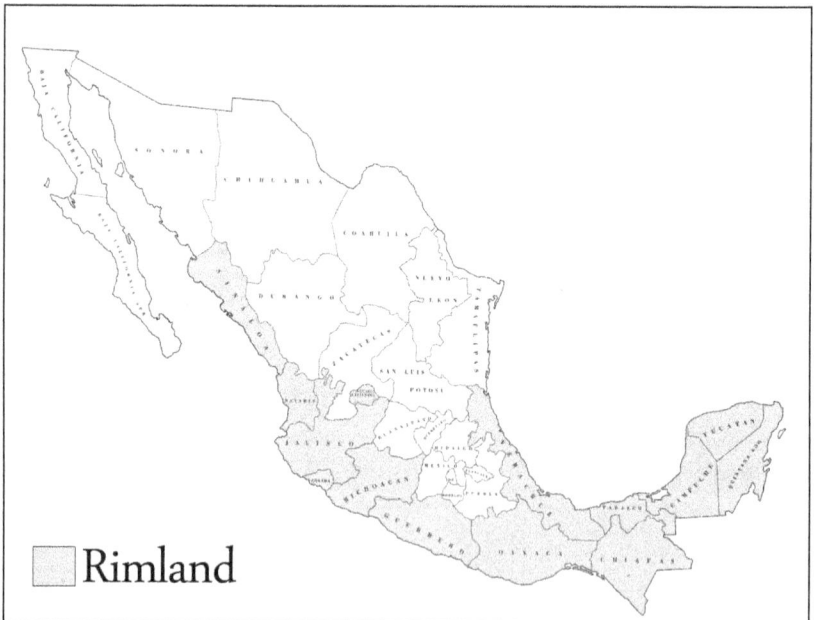

Rimland

MAP 3 Courtesy of the U.S. Army War College; used with permission.

Three major cartels began in rimland states: LFM/LCT, Sinaloa, and BLO. These rimland cartels have used the strategies of brute force, denial, deterrence, and punishment to deal with external challenges and internal fractures and to extend their influence into other areas. But due to their distance from plazas, rimland cartels have had special challenges that make the use of their corporate logic more understandable. The large physical range of their operations means that the number and the complexity of disputes increase because it is more difficult to oversee transactions and exact a cut from each of them.[15]

Criminals in the underworld, as individuals in the overworld, might develop relations of trust and reciprocity that escape the mafia as the guarantor of transactions, thus bypassing it. Such an overstretched mafia would need to rely on an army of enforcers able to intervene in troublesome spots around the country, protecting the "legitimate" representative of the organization, in ways that do not differ significantly from sending troops to crush a rebellion in a breakaway region.[16]

This is precisely what is happening in cities like Juarez where rimland cartels must constantly reinforce their ranks with gangs who are used to enforce their will against local groups who resist the "invaders."

LFM began in the rimland state of Michoacán; due to its ability to control the port city of Lazaro Cardenas, the cartel was able to control a major smuggling node. The port accepts more cargo than the twenty-one other ports in Mexico and lies within two hundred miles of half the Mexican population.[17] The transit routes that radiate from the port are an essential part of the heroin, cocaine, and meth smuggling infrastructure in the rimland. Without having an active presence in the heartland to access the plazas, LFM gradually expanded into other rimland states of Guerrero, Colima, Jalisco and the nearby peripheral states of Guanajuato, Morelos, Queretaro, and Mexico, violently evicting other crime groups in an effort to enhance its position in relation to other major cartels.[18] LFM previously negotiated for access to plazas, but its alliance with the Gulf and Sinaloa cartels in the New Federation against Los Zetas may be seen as a way to guarantee some LFM presence in the heartland. However, LCT's seeming alliance with Los Zetas appears to be merely a way to mop up LFM remnants in the rimland.

The Sinaloa cartel is based in the city of Culiacan. Its rimland location also permitted the cartel to extend its influence from its proximity to port cities. It controls the ports of Mazatlan, Manzanillo, and Puerto Vallarta. It was also able to extend itself in the heartland state of Sonora with the assistance of its one-time allies, the BLO. The Sinaloa cartel is the first rimland cartel that has sought to extend its presence by battling with heartland cartels. Because the state of Sinaloa is five hundred miles from the U.S. border, the cartel requires some sort of accommodation or presence in the heartland. This explains its actions to support a faction of the Tijuana cartel and its all-out assault against the Juarez cartel. But with the states of Sonora and Chihuahua bordering Sinaloa, in combination with the remote and rugged terrain, the Sinaloa cartel can secure itself in its rural base and support their operations in other areas.[19] The city of Culiacan also figures prominently in narco-cultura—the figure known as Jesús Malverde is said to have originated in this area, and the shrine to him is near the old statehouse in Culiacan and is regularly visited by a number of devotees.[20] Equally significant is the belief among local residents that drugs are integral to their way of life. One street vendor said that "the economy of Culiacan is half tomatoes . . . and half marijuana. If they are really going to fight the narcos here, the economy of the state will completely collapse."[21] Such a sentiment shows how soft power of the Sinaloa cartel is generated and how it is able to gain community acquiescence in the area of its origin.

BLO also has its genesis in the rimland state of Sinaloa, having once been aligned with the Sinaloa cartel in the Federacion. The BLO was able to secure routes in Jalisco, Michoacán, Guerrero, and Morelos to smuggle cocaine.[22] The Sinaloa-BLO split and the intracartel split in the BLO brought high levels of violence in the state of Sinaloa. In early 2010, the BLO, in league with Los Zetas, were involved in a war against the New Federation of the Gulf cartel, Sinaloa cartel, and LFM in the heartland city of Reynosa, Tamaulipas.

The rimland states have also been subjected to violent designs of heartland cartels to control these critical nodes in the drug trafficking chain. Cartels based in the heartland have not ignored rimland territories nor have they relied on alliances with rimland-based cartels. The Gulf cartel has battled the Sinaloa cartel in the southernmost states of the rimland, but their alliance along with LFM as the New Federation has shifted the bulk of their attention to attacking Los Zetas in the heartland state of Tamaulipas. In the Tierra Caliente region, which is at the intersection of Michoacán, Guerrero, and Mexico state, LFM battled Los Zetas when they were linked with the Gulf cartel for control of crop areas and transit routes.[23] Vacancy chains in the rimland have led to violence between these groups after Los Zetas split with the Gulf cartel. With the 2010 death of Sinaloa leader Ignacio Coronel Villarreal, who was in control of Colima, Los Zetas and LFM fought to take over his operations.

Guatemala's proximity to the rimland states of Chiapas and Campeche has been an operational benefit for Los Zetas. Through their association with Guatemalan former special forces, Los Zetas have been able to smuggle cocaine and heroin overland across the border, set up training camps in Guatemalan territory, and evade rivals and the Mexican government. This access to a unique part of the rimland has enabled Los Zetas to maintain themselves against the assaults from the government and the New Federation in the heartland region.

The Periphery

The remaining states are peripheral areas that are not as consequential to the movement and production of drugs but contain small retail markets, produce some drugs, and serve as refuges for top cartel leaders (see map 4). While some cities and towns in the heartland and rimland also contain retail markets, their primary importance is to supply the main market in the United States. Some violence in the rimland, however, is for access to peripheral markets. Much of the fighting between the BLO factions, Los Zetas, and LFM/LCT in the states of Guerrero, Morelos, and Hidalgo are over the control of the flow of drugs into the Mexico City market.[24] The periphery

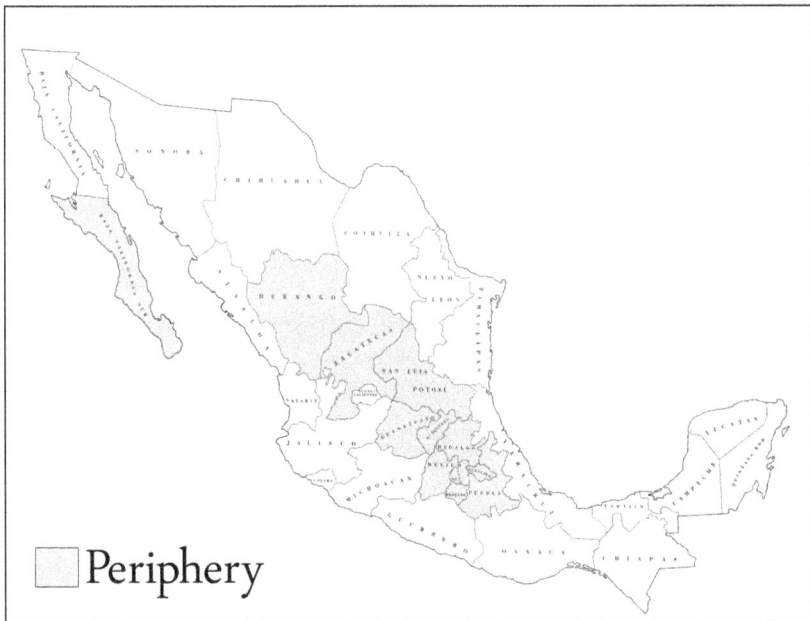

Periphery

MAP 4 Courtesy of the U.S. Army War College; used with permission.

has a subsidiary value but still serves a function in geo-criminality. The periphery does not merit the same application of corporate logic or the strategies of violence given the low stakes in this area.

Mexico City and much of the country's central and southern interior are not as subject to the same intensity of disputes in the heartland and rimland that occur among the major cartels.[25] The periphery has not been immune to cartel violence; there have been a number of instances of kidnappings and murders but on a much lower scale than in many states in the heartland and rimland. For example, in the state of Baja California Sur, there was only one drug-related death in 2010. One explanation for lower levels of violence, other than the relative lack of significance of many areas in the periphery to the movement or production of drugs, is that the "corporate offices" of the cartels are located in this region.[26] In these areas, cartel leaders have attempted to create safe havens. With the help of complicit state agents, the major cartel leaders were largely kept safely away from the threat of arrest and extradition before 2006.

After 2006, safe havens have become more complex. The capital of Mexico City represents an example of this complexity. The capital has been largely a place of peace where high-level drug traffickers coexist with each other and the government. As William Finnegan put it, the capital is a place in "which no single syndicate can control but where every self-respecting cartel must be represented."[27] But the periphery as a site of refuge has been under challenge. This is evident in the number of high-level drug cartel members who have been arrested or killed within this region. The sons of the leaders of the Sinaloa and Gulf cartels were caught in the upscale suburbs of Mexico City; Edgar Valdez Villarreal of the BLO was caught in Morelos near Mexico City; Teodoro Garcia Simental of the Tijuana cartel was caught in Los Cabos, Baja California Sur; and Arturo Beltrán Leyva was killed in a town in the state of Morelos. Law enforcement officials have also been targeted. In 2008 alone, three senior law enforcement officials were assassinated: Roberto Bravo, Director of Investigations of the Sensitive Investigations Unit of the Federal Police; Edgar Gomez, General Coordinator for Regional Security at the Mexican Secretariat of Public Security; and Igor Calderón of the Federal Investigative Agency. Nonetheless, government corruption still provides a degree of safety in some cases. A day before the arrest of a Mexican police officer, he received a call on his cellphone, warning him that he was about to be arrested. The phone call was traced back to the offices of the federal police in Mexico City.[28]

The wealthier suburbs in the heartland city of Monterrey, Nuevo Leon, served as a type of hideout for some of Mexico's biggest drug lords, particularly Los Zetas.[29]

Once considered off-limits by rival gangs, Monterrey experienced a sharp uptick in criminal violence such as extortion, carjacking, kidnapping, and armed robbery due to its geographic position as the side of the triangle that links it with Reynosa. But with attacks against drug trafficking nodes having increasingly taken their toll, several gangs and cartels have shifted their focus to these ancillary crimes as a way to compensate for a loss in income. This new wave of crime and violence has forced many top leaders to move around to various other cities in the periphery in the search for greater sanctuary.

The state of Durango is a unique peripheral state. On the map, Durango appears as a type of hub upon which many states with key trafficking nodes swivel. It lies at the intersection of several rimland states, key heartland states, and the northern tip of the interior periphery. As a consequence, Durango's hub nature has meant both that it is a location of violence and that it radiates violence to other states. The outbreak of violence in Durango in 2009 was dramatic—a nearly 600 percent increase over the previous year.[30] Most of the violence was due to the invasion of the Gulf cartel and its then enforcers, Los Zetas, to challenge the Sinaloa leader Joaquin Guzman on a formerly quiet patch of his home turf where many believe he has been living.[31] Reflecting its hub nature, Durango is also the location of Gomez Palacio Prison, where authorities released inmates at night to commit contract killings in the city of Torreon in the neighboring heartland state of Coahuila.

The pressure exerted against Los Zetas in the heartland bodes ill for parts of the periphery. Sustained attacks against the group have led to fighting between its gangs and LFM/LCT and other gangs in Mexico City to control retail sales. This is a possible omen that points to the effects of intense fighting in the heartland and the rimland—the periphery is likely to be swept up in violence as groups begin to use it as an area to retreat and regroup while simultaneously attempting to muscle in on previously peaceful local drug markets.

Geo-Criminality and High-Intensity Crime

Geo-criminality demonstrates the mosaic quality of the cartel wars in Mexico by explaining the reasons why violence has occurred in many locations but has not engulfed all of Mexico. The combination of the five laws of corporate logic, other cultural and political drivers of violence, alliance-building activities, and the strategic use of violence makes geo-criminality another way that high-intensity crime, rather than low-intensity conflict, is a better way to explain Mexico's mosaic cartel war. The cartels view the locations where they carry out violence as essential because of the locations' importance for money making rather than policymaking. Their explicit commercial motive is only incidentally a political motive.

The targets of cartel violence in these regions, although similar in type to those that would be selected by insurgents and terrorists, are directly related to their place in the drug trafficking network as expressed by geo-criminality. More police, mayors, and state agents have been killed in the heartland and rimland, reflecting plomo of the cartels' corporate logic (see graph 1).

What has been missing from these statistics is the number of municipal police that have been intimidated into leaving their jobs by the cartels. For example, the entire fourteen-member police force of a rural community nearly forty miles away from Monterrey in Nuevo Leon resigned after their headquarters was attacked with assault rifles and grenades in October 2010. In another instance, a twenty-year-old

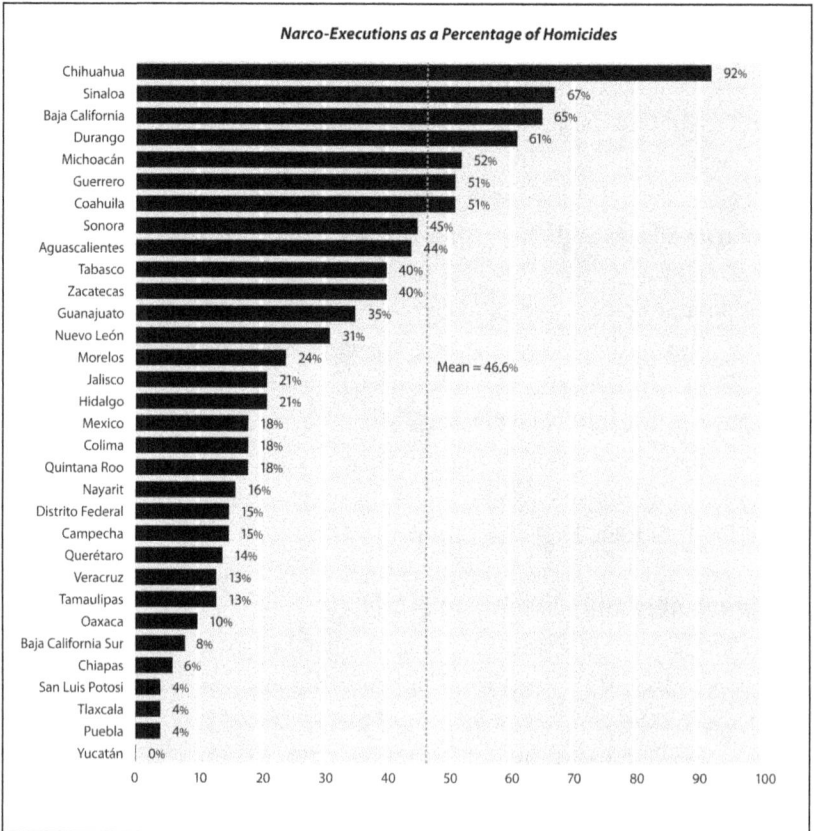

Narco-Executions as a Percentage of Homicides

State	Percentage
Chihuahua	92%
Sinaloa	67%
Baja California	65%
Durango	61%
Michoacán	52%
Guerrero	51%
Coahuila	51%
Sonora	45%
Aguascalientes	44%
Tabasco	40%
Zacatecas	40%
Guanajuato	35%
Nuevo León	31%
Morelos	24%
Jalisco	21%
Hidalgo	21%
Mexico	18%
Colima	18%
Quintana Roo	18%
Nayarit	16%
Distrito Federal	15%
Campecha	15%
Querétaro	14%
Veracruz	13%
Tamaulipas	13%
Oaxaca	10%
Baja California Sur	8%
Chiapas	6%
San Luis Potosi	4%
Tlaxcala	4%
Puebla	4%
Yucatán	0%

Mean = 46.6%

GRAPH 1 Compiled by Diego Valle-Jones

college student became the chief of police in a town outside of Juarez when no other candidates accepted the position.

The killings of mayors also fit the pattern of deaths of state agents. Since 2006, over a dozen mayors have been killed, mirroring the patterns of geo-criminality. Three were from Chihuahua, two from Tamaulipas, two from Michoacán, two from Nuevo Leon, two from Oaxaca, two from Durango, one from Guerrero, and one from San Luis Potosi.[32]

More journalists have also been killed in the heartland, demonstrating the cartels' desire to operate in the shadows. Particularly hard hit was Tamaulipas, which was ranked first in the number of disappeared journalists in 2010.[33] The Gulf cartel has not only matched Los Zetas's more brutal tactics against the media but has augmented its influence by sending checks to reporters for favorable coverage and sending "spokesmen" to crime scenes to dictate angles for news stories.[34] The struggle among the warring cartels to control information began in tandem with a type of cartel blitzkrieg that occurred in that city.

The overall rates of homicides attributed to cartel violence reflect the importance that the cartels place on the heartland and rimland. In 2008, the six municipalities with the highest homicide rates were in the heartland: Juarez, Nogales, Hidalgo de Parral, Chihuahua, Tijuana, and Tecate. By 2010, Chihuahua and the rimland state of Sinaloa represented 45 percent of all homicides, followed by Guerrero, Tamaulipas, Durango, and Baja California.[35] The percentage of homicides attributed to cartels, known as narco-executions, shows the pattern even more clearly—the highest rates are in the heartland, followed by those in the rimland. However, once again the exception is the peripheral state of Durango (see graph 2).

From the pattern of killings in Mexico, the geo-criminal factors of the mosaic war become clearer and shed light on the behavior of the cartels. Heartland cartels have had difficulty in seeking to seize and control rimland territory in order to take over ports and transit areas where drugs make their way to the heartland. Rimland cartels cannot simply shut off the supply of drugs to the heartland as a way to exert pressure on heartland cartels; rimland cartels must either make deals with heartland cartels or attempt violent takeovers of plazas in the heartland. Heartland cartels can, on the other hand, negotiate the prices for drugs transported from or through rimland territory. Once again, trust has often broken down, leading violent entrepreneurs to resort to their core competency—the use of violence. Machismo explains why many cartels and gangs, when confronted on their home turf, have refused to capitulate and have continued to fight, adding to the body count in places like Juarez and Reynosa.

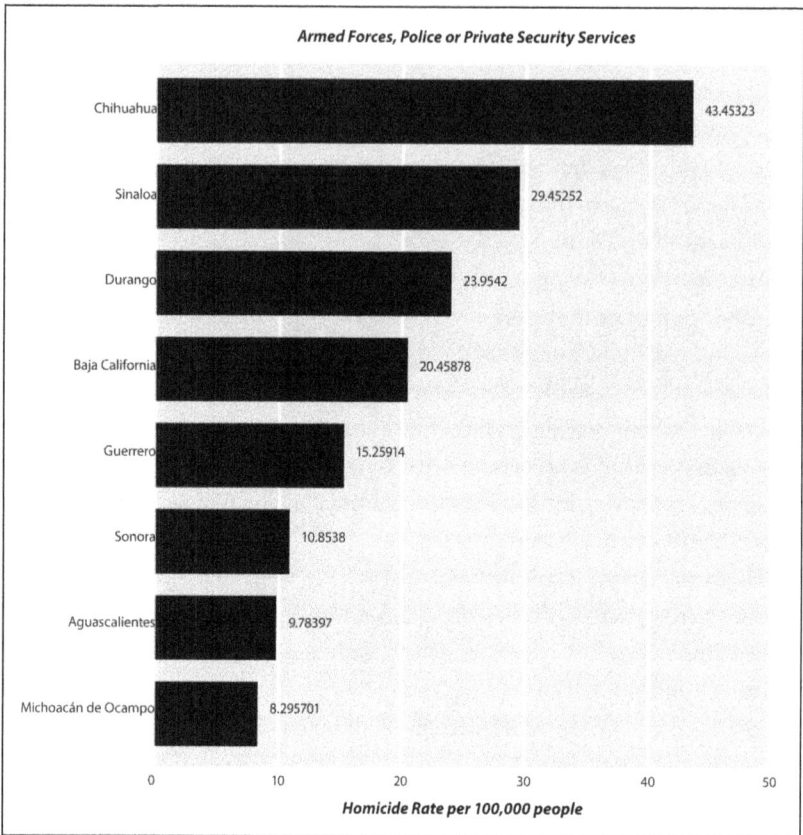

Armed Forces, Police or Private Security Services

State	Homicide Rate per 100,000 people
Chihuahua	43.45323
Sinaloa	29.45252
Durango	23.9542
Baja California	20.45878
Guerrero	15.25914
Sonora	10.8538
Aguascalientes	9.78397
Michoacán de Ocampo	8.295701

GRAPH 2   Compiled by Diego Valle-Jones

Violence in the rimland has been largely due to intracartel strife and splits, while attacks by heartland cartels in the rimland have been punitive expeditions against rimland cartels as revenge for their actions in the heartland or for reneging on agreements. The arrests and killings of kingpins by the government have mainly occurred in areas of the periphery; the arrests and killings of members of the BLO in the periphery are likely due to having been pushed out of Sinaloa because of its split with the Sinaloa cartel. However, the peripheral state of Durango has been a site of violence between heartland and rimland cartels due to its unique hub quality. In some ways, Durango is a microcosm of geo-criminality and of Mexico's mosaic war.

The lower incidents of homicides among state agents in the periphery reflect the use of plata to gain the acquiescence of local authorities. The existence of corruption is another element that separates high-intensity crime from low-intensity conflict. The best example of this distinction is Mexico City and other neighboring areas of the periphery. Known high-level cartel members live in and work from this area with the knowledge and complicity of Mexican authorities. In this area of the periphery, cartel leaders and government officials are, in many respects, colleagues rather than adversaries. This accommodation on both sides is the result of the economic imperatives of the drug trade rather than political calculations of terrorists or insurgents.

Geo-Criminality and the United States

Mexico's capacity gaps and functional holes are more apparent when viewed through the lens of geo-criminality. The hypercompetitive illegal market extends throughout Mexico, but various states fulfill different purposes for the cartels. The territory of Mexico is permeated and carved up by the profit-seeking motivations of cartels. The extraordinary level of violence and corruption that diminishes the competence and legitimacy of the Mexican state is located in a number of heartland and rimland states. The periphery, in many respects, exists only because of the Mexican government's corruption.

The demand side of the hypercompetitive illegal market lies over the border in the United States. This means that the effects of geo-criminality also extend northward and cannot be separated from cartel strategies. The effects have been mild when placed in comparison to the violence and insecurity that have been experienced in numerous areas of Mexico. Nonetheless, criminality that emanates across a border often begins to erode national welfare before it becomes a threat to national security.[36] The blurring line between the two is the subject of the next chapter.

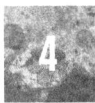

THE SPREAD
The Effects on the United States

High-intensity crime has not broken out in the United States as a result of the mosaic cartel war in Mexico, but its occurrence in Mexico has affected the United States nonetheless. The perniciousness of the hypercompetitive illegal market encompasses the United States, and the corporate logic of the cartels challenges a number of U.S. national interests. The geographic proximity of the two countries cannot help but cast the shadow of geo-criminality upon the United States. The nearly two-thousand-mile-long border is crossed by 250 million counted people per year. "It spans four U.S. states, six Mexican states, twenty railroad crossings, and there are about thirty city pairings along it (United States and Mexican cities directly across from each other). About 12 million people live on both sides."[1] Mexico is the third-largest U.S. trading partner and the third-largest supplier of crude oil and constitutes bilateral trade equaling $350 billion annually.[2] And, with a population of over 100 million, Mexico and its mosaic cartel war are of acute concern to the United States.

The connections between the United States and Mexico cannot be underestimated, nor can the possible dangers that such connections can generate. Eighty-seven percent of items manufactured in Mexican maquiladoras come from the six states in the geo-criminal heartland of the cartels; 85 percent of all trade between the United States and Mexico passes through the heartland, and as seen in the previous chapter, the majority of drug killings have occurred in this same region. Cartels by their nature as violent entrepreneurs exercise their corporate logic in ways that undermine civil society, destabilize governmental institutions and processes, and erode the rule of law.[3] Because this activity takes place in the cities and states of the geo-criminal heartland, U.S. interests in maintaining a Mexico that is secure and contributes to U.S. prosperity are jeopardized. As mentioned in chapter 1, President Obama's *National Security Strategy* emphasized the stability and security in Mexico as indispensable. This is the first *National Security Strategy* to use the words "stability and security" in conjunction with Mexico. Significant increases of instability and insecurity along the border of the world's only superpower—one that has assumed dominance of North America and control of its borders—would create the potential for serious repercussions.[4]

The United States is already experiencing the effects of weakening stability and security in Mexico created by the mosaic cartel war. These effects can be placed under three broad categories. First, there are spillover effects that occur in the United States that are directly related to drug crimes committed by cartels, gangs, and drug users. Second, there are also spill-back effects that damage U.S. interests in Mexico. Finally, there are spill-around effects that challenge U.S. interests in the region and around the world. All of these reflect how far-reaching and widespread Mexico's high-intensity crime has become.

Spillover Effects in the United States

The spillover effects present high stakes for the United States. Security of citizenry and territory are the sine qua non of sovereignty, and spillover effects challenge this basic responsibility of the state. Because the main demand of the hypercompetitive illegal market lies in the United States, cartels as violent entrepreneurs cannot help but apply a degree of their corporate logic within its borders. Cartels and gangs that operate in the United States attempt to adhere closely to the law of corporate logic that emphasizes the use of purposeful and directed violence because "Mexican trafficking organizations understand that intentional targeting of U.S. persons or interests unrelated to the drug trade would likely undermine their own business interests."[5] In fact, an August 2010 report by the Congressional Research Service that focused specifically on the issue of spillover violence found that there is no publicly available data that can "determine the proportion of violent crimes that are related to drug trafficking or, even more specifically, the proportion of drug trafficking–related violent crimes that are attributable to spillover violence."[6] This does not mean that there has not been any spillover violence, but that disaggregating the data from sources such as the FBI's Uniform Crime Report is exceptionally thorny. Simply put, this means that violent crimes attributable to Mexican drug trafficking have occurred, but measuring them in the aggregate has been difficult. Nonetheless, the spillover effects do not solely include violence. As seen in chapter 2, a cartel's actions are more than the threat or application of violence. Therefore, spillover effects are more than just acts of violence but are related to the activities of cartels and their gang affiliates that negatively affect citizens, military, law enforcement, government institutions, and private businesses.[7]

The pattern of spillover effects follows the flow of drugs from the Mexican geo-criminal heartland states to the numerous retail markets in the United States as well as the flow of guns and money southbound. To move drugs into the United States from Mexico, cartels must circumvent, co-opt, or confront law enforcement. Circumvention occurs when drugs are clandestinely transported across the border. It is common for smugglers to hide drugs in vehicles—cars, trucks, buses, trains—and on their person and to use people who routinely cross the border each day. Cartels have also used aircraft, including ultralights, to smuggle drugs; moved them through sophisticated tunnels under the border; and used semisubmersible vessels. The Tijuana cartel has used small boats to drop off drug loads as well as migrants along the beaches of San Diego County.[8] U.S. law enforcement has also been subjected to plata o plomo approaches, but to a lesser degree than seen in Mexico. The sheer number of federal law enforcement agents who have been prosecuted for bribery shows how far corruption can reach. According to the FBI, there have been 400 public corruption cases originating from the U.S.-Mexico border region; in the 2009 fiscal year there were more than 100 arrests and about 130 state and federal cases prosecuted.[9] From 2004 to 2010, 103 Customs and Border Protection (CBP) officers have been arrested or indicted on corruption charges.[10] The 2009 arrest of Richard Padilla Cramer, a high-ranking official in U.S. Immigration and Customs Enforcement (ICE), shows that not only front-line law enforcement officials are subjected to enticement of the cartels; top officials have been lured into assisting the cartels move drugs. Cramer was arrested for helping a Mexican cartel move drugs, advising traffickers on law enforcement tactics, and pulling secret files to help them identify turncoats.[11] Perhaps more troubling is the desire of Mexican cartels to infiltrate U.S. law enforcement by placing their own personnel in its agencies. James Tomsheck, the assistant commissioner for internal affairs at CBP, has stated that "there have been verifiable instances where people were directed to CBP to apply for positions only for the purpose of enhancing the goals of criminal organizations. They had been selected because they had no criminal record; a background investigation would not develop derogatory information."[12]

Law enforcement officers near the border have also been subjected to violence and intimidation directed by gangs and cartels as ways to ensure that drug loads reach their destinations. U.S. law enforcement personnel along the border have been assaulted by rocks, guns, Molotov cocktails, and vehicles. Border Patrol agents have been attacked while giving chase to vehicles laden with drugs.[13] Attacks on law enforcement agents are "often intended to deter them from seizing illicit drug shipments or used as a diversion to smuggle drug shipments."[14] The U.S. Department of Homeland Security (DHS) sent out a memo warning Border Patrol agents that they could now become targets of hired assassins as retaliation for tighter border security.[15] Local law enforcement officers have received threats from cartels not to intercept drug loads under penalty of death.[16] In a 2010 incident, a Border Patrol agent was killed when his team encountered a "rip crew" of five men near a national park in Arizona.[17] "Rip crews" are organized to rob drug smugglers as they travel along their route.

The Mexican military has also been accused of crossing into California, Arizona, and Texas to protect drug loads.[18] The number of incursions by Mexican security officials has been steadily rising. A recent analysis by Judicial Watch of data from U.S. Customs and Border Protection showed:

- 76 Mexican government incursions from January 2008 to December 2009 (data missing from February 2009)
- 50 Mexican government incursions in 2008, double the number of incursions from the previous year
- 528 assaults against CBP agents from January to June 2008
- 11 assaults against National Guard agents with CBP from January to June 2008[19]

Most strikingly, an unmanned aerial vehicle, or drone, owned by the Mexican government crashed in the backyard of an El Paso, Texas, home in late 2010.[20] Up to that date, it was not known that the Mexican government was using drones along the border.

It is not only law enforcement officials who have been attacked near the border. U.S. citizens have also been victimized. A rancher along the Arizona-Sonora border, Robert Krentz, was killed on his land in April 2010 by a person who is widely believed to have been either drug smuggler or migrant escort.[21] Falcon Lake, straddling Texas and Tamaulipas, has been the site of piracy conducted against Americans by Los Zetas. The area around the lake is lucrative smuggling territory; the Border Patrol seized a total of $14 million worth of marijuana in 2009.[22] With the pressure exerted on them by the New Federation and the Mexican military, Los Zetas have been forced to diversify their crimes in order to earn money. Using high-powered boats and brandishing weapons, Los Zetas have ambushed fishermen and tourists who have strayed into the Mexican side of Falcon Lake, demanding money, weapons, and drugs.[23] The importance of holding the lake for Los Zetas became clear when the first violent fatality occurred in September 2010. A Jet Skier was killed by

Los Zetas, who possibly mistook him and his wife for Gulf cartel members intruding in Los Zetas's territory.[24] The ramifications were felt in Tamaulipas; the lead investigator was decapitated, and his head was delivered in a suitcase to the Mexican military.[25] Such violence also negatively affects the local economy of the Falcon Lake area, which is linked to recreational activities; many regular and potential visitors have been too frightened to come to Falcon Lake.[26]

Areas that straddle the border and that are difficult to monitor make them prime locations for the transportation of drugs. Along with tributaries, deserts that reach over both sides of the border are used by cartels and present threats to U.S. citizens. The Buenos Aires National Wildlife Refuge is nearly in the center of Arizona's border with Mexico; part of it has been closed to the U.S. public because of "adverse effects of border-related activity." The public notice of the closure read in part:

The U.S. Fish and Wildlife Service has closed a portion of the Buenos Aires National Wildlife Refuge. . . . This area is about 3,500 acres in size. . . . The international border with Mexico has become increasingly violent. Assaults on law enforcement officers and violence against migrants have escalated. Violence on the Refuge associated with smugglers and border bandits has been well-documented.[27]

Even federal lands far from the border have been penetrated by cartels and gangs. Mexican gang members with links to the cartels have been found to be growing marijuana in U.S. national parks. In Sequoia National Park, authorities found marijuana crops worth $40 million being grown far off well-traveled trails. Along with the marijuana, authorities arrested thirty-eight people and seized twenty-nine automatic weapons, high-powered rifles, and other guns.[28] The U.S. Forest Service has discovered pot farms in sixty-one national forests across sixteen states in 2009.[29] Seven hundred so-called grow sites were discovered on U.S. Forest Service land in California alone in 2007 and 2008.[30] The use of these areas for drug cultivation and production has damaged fragile ecosystems with the use of pesticides, chemicals, and the discarding of refuse and human waste. Camps are set up by traffickers, and it is estimated that they produce about eight pounds per person per day in refuse and human waste alone. Violence has also come to parks. A U.S. Park Service ranger in Arizona's Organ Pipe Cactus National Monument was gunned down by a Mexican pot smuggler in August 2002. Gangs from Mexico have also been found to be exploiting the land on Indian reservations. One grow site in Washington State's Yakama Reservation featured a makeshift shrine to Jesús Malverde.[31]

Growing and producing drugs in the United States, rather than relying on conducting these activities solely in Mexico, is another way for cartels to circumvent tougher border enforcement activities. All of these activities affect the ability of the U.S. public to enjoy these areas for recreation, to preserve the parks for future generations of visitors, and to protect the ecology of these lands.

Because of activities along the border and on federal lands, Internet and media rumors often appear plausible. In July 2010, the Internet was abuzz with a story that Los Zetas had seized two ranches in Laredo, Texas.[32] This story was proven false. Similarly, Arizona governor Jan Brewer was forced to admit that she was mistaken in her claim that beheadings by drug cartels and migrant smugglers were occurring in the desert. Such rumors often require law enforcement to investigate their validity, creating distractions of time and resources that could be spent on actual cases.

Along with violence, intimidation, and corruption associated with the movement of drugs from plazas across the border, other visible crimes have been associated with wholesale and retail sales of narcotics in the United States. Once in the United States, drugs are transported by smugglers and gangs along major U.S. highways.

Interstate 10 as well as Interstates 8 and 20 are among those most used by drug couriers, as evidenced by drug seizure data showing that from 2008 through October 2009, nearly 19 percent of all reported interstate cocaine seizures and 7 percent of all reported interstate heroin seizures occurred on these routes. . . . Interstates 15, 80, 70, and 40 are [also] leading routes, and seizures on these interstates accounted for 46 percent of all reported methamphetamine seizures and 31 percent of all marijuana seizures on interstates from 2008 through October 2009.[33]

Via these routes, drugs arrive at a few major U.S. drug markets where there are large drug user populations and where drugs are further distributed to smaller markets. The main destinations are Chicago, Denver, Detroit, Houston, Miami, New York, and Tucson.[34] Gangs facilitate the movement of illicit drugs to urban, suburban, and rural areas of the United States for distribution and sale. Armed convoys have been employed to protect drug loads along highways.[35] Gangs also aid in the movement of hard currency and weapons to Mexico, as well as enforce the collection of drug profits. According to the National Drug Intelligence Center, gang affiliates of the cartels—street gangs, prison gangs, and outlaw motorcycle gangs—have a presence in approximately 230 U.S. cities.[36]

A portion of the spillover effects in the United States is closely related to the demand side of the equation. Crime in demand markets usually involves disputes over sales, territory, inventory, and profits; crimes against people and property by drug users to pay for their drugs; and crimes perpetrated by those under the influence of illicit narcotics.[37] By one estimate, a heroin user commits two hundred crimes a year in order to supply his or her habit.[38] According to another study, meth abusers regularly commit identity theft to acquire funds to pay for their addiction.[39] Grisly crimes against those associated with Mexican drug trafficking have occurred in a number of cities far from the border but along major transit routes or in distribution cities. In Birmingham, Alabama, five men were found with their throats slit in 2009 over a drug debt of $400,000; Atlanta police found a man beaten, bound, gagged, and chained to a wall over a $300,000 debt owed to the Gulf cartel.[40] Beheadings in Mexico were steadily moving in a northward direction, with some cases reportedly crossing the border and occurring in the United States.[41] The exact number of beheadings and those linked to cartels is not known because many police departments do not report them out of concern that media stories might frighten residents and give their municipalities a bad reputation. In fact, the first confirmed and acknowledged beheading in the United States that was linked to Mexican drug trafficking occurred in October 2010 but was not publicly verified until March 2011.[42]

Beyond acts of violence along the border, on federal lands, or in retail markets, some of the violence in the United States is an extension of cartel disputes in Mexico. Home invasions and kidnappings in Phoenix are an example of this extension. Far from being random victims of gangs and cartels, those who have been beaten, kidnapped, and killed were swept up in the corporate logic of the cartels. They have been victims particularly of laws one and two of a cartel's corporate logic—the spurring of new markets and the use of purposeful, directed violence against rivals and traitors. Gang members have been hired by cartels to kidnap or kill rival cartel or gang members, the relatives of rival cartel members, and those who have split from the group and their relatives. These acts are meant to demonstrate the reach of the cartel and therefore to coerce rivals and traitors. Some kidnappings are conducted to get money from those who owe money to cartels. That these acts are aimed at those who are involved in trafficking or who are related to drug traffickers should not be seen as a consolation. Portraying these people as somehow deserving their fate belies respect for the rule of law and assumes that innocents are not harmed in the commission of these crimes.[43] In one incident, a Mexican drug gang impersonated law enforcement SWAT members to gain access to residences of their targets; over one hundred rounds were fired in a residential neighborhood by the perpetrators, endangering a number of innocent lives.[44]

The spillover effects occur not only along the northbound drug trafficking network. The southbound gun trade contributes to the means that cartels and gangs in Mexico use to raise the intensity of violence. The illegal gun trade is another spillover effect that is part of the hypercompetitive illegal market of drug trafficking; smuggled weapons can fetch a price 300 percent higher than their legal market value.[45] Lucrative profit and the heavy restrictions on purchasing and owning firearms in Mexico, combined with a demand for weapons, has created conditions for crimes that break federal firearms laws. Many of the weapons used by Mexican drug cartels are purchased at American gun shows or gun shops. "Straw purchasers"—American citizens who have clean criminal records that can pass background checks—are paid by Mexican gang members to buy guns on their behalf. With many family members residing in the United States, Mexican residents can ask them to purchase a weapon on their behalf. A Houston gun dealer, for example, was recruited by his cousin to sell weapons to Los Zetas.[46] Firearms dealers in the United States have also been enticed into breaking laws to earn extra money by supplying guns directly to gangs.[47] In some instances, gangs not only use straw purchasers but resort to thefts and robberies of U.S. firearm shops along the border.[48] The guns are then smuggled back into Mexico. With repeated trips across the border, called "ant runs," smugglers are able to keep Mexican cartels and gangs well stocked with weapons.

The use of U.S. citizens as straw purchasers and the crimes of U.S. gun shop owners points to another spillover effect that is especially pernicious—the luring of American citizens into committing crimes that assist Mexican cartels and gangs. The 2009 National Gang Threat Assessment from the U.S. Department of Justice identified a number of Mexican gangs like Barrio Azteca, Surenos, and La Eme whose members were also serving in the U.S. military. In 2009, an active duty U.S. Army soldier was accused of carrying out a hit against a cartel informant at the direction of a Mexican cartel.[49] Such infiltration is significant because "gang members with military training pose a unique threat to law enforcement personnel because of the distinctive military skills that they possess and their willingness to teach these skills to fellow gang members."[50] The penetration of the U.S. armed services by gang members and those willing to carry out the orders of cartels represents a deterioration of national loyalty that is a core military value.

Infiltration by gangs and cartels points to an additional spillover effect of cartels' corporate logic, namely the pervasiveness of cartel soft power along with the unique narco-cultura of Mexican crime. Some young Americans are drawn to the way of life that is offered by cartels and gangs because it appears to offer them empowerment. From the impoverished neighborhoods of U.S. border towns, some teenagers have been recruited to conduct crimes on behalf of cartels and gangs. In late 2010, a fourteen-year-old American boy was captured in Mexico and accused of being a hit man (namely decapitating four people) for the BLO.[51] In a phenomenon very similar to what occurs in Mexico, the cartels seduce teenagers and young people by waving "power, cash, cars, easy money. And, these kids all have that romantic notion they are going to live forever."[52] Narcocorridos are often just as popular in some U.S. Mexican communities. Teens have also become involved in the worship of narco-saints; in one incident, the teen killers collected their victims' blood in a glass and toasted Santa Muerte.[53] The evangelical nature of LFM and its successor, LCT, has also crossed the border. Before its rebranding as LCT, a considerable number of LFM members had been arrested in the United States, including the largest U.S. law enforcement sting, which netted over three hundred members of the organization.

In the final stage of the drug trafficking process, collecting and moving profit, the United States has also been affected by Mexican cartels. Cartels have laundered money through U.S. financial institutions. HSBC, Wachovia, and Bank of America admitted to failing to properly monitor money transfers. Federal agents caught people who worked for Mexican cartels depositing illicit funds in Bank of America accounts in Atlanta, Chicago, and Brownsville, Texas, from 2002 to 2009. Wachovia admitted that it failed to monitor and report suspected money laundering activities to the tune of $110 million, including funds that were used to purchase four planes that were used to smuggle twenty-two tons of cocaine into the United States.[54] The movement of hard currency back to Mexico is another related spillover effect. According to U.S. Customs and Border Protection, $44 million was seized between late 2008 and early 2010 during inspections of vehicles and people leaving the United States for Mexico at U.S. border ports.[55] The cash is moved to Mexico similar to the way drugs are brought across northbound—U.S. cities near the border or that contain lucrative retail markets act as collection points for cash. "Stash houses" are used to break down the hard currency into loads that can be moved in vehicles or carried by individuals across to Mexico. One tactic of currency smugglers is to "clone" vehicles to make them look like Border Patrol or local law enforcement vehicles that can then attempt to enter restricted areas near the border to transfer loads of currency to waiting partners on the Mexican side.[56] Using law enforcement or emergency vehicles "is a security risk."[57] Smugglers have even used fake uniforms to impersonate law enforcement as a way to complete the ruse.[58]

Some of the spillover effects are unrelated to the movement of drugs, guns, or profit. The entry of cartels into migrant smuggling has also complicated U.S. immigration enforcement as well. What was once an industry run by individual migrant smugglers, or coyotes, is now in the purview of the cartels, which have more sophisticated techniques. Migrants who are smuggled by cartels "now face even higher incidents of physical abuse and rape, extortion for additional sums of money, or ending up as indentured household servants or forced into prostitution."[59] Such victimization, when discovered by law enforcement, requires investigation and resources to deal with those who have suffered abuse. An additional complication created by the involvement of drug cartels in human smuggling is their capacity to assist in the hundreds of illegal border crossings of people from special-interest countries like China, Iraq, Iran, Afghanistan, and Pakistan. Reportedly, some alien smuggling organizations and Mexican cartels specialize in smuggling special-interest aliens into the United States.[60] "Gangs' most significant potential contribution to terrorism within the United States, though, is probably not direct association but by infiltrating terrorists into the U.S. and providing opportunities for them to conduct reconnaissance and attacks."[61] As a result, individuals from these countries who are caught require more screening and processing to determine their exact intentions for crossing into U.S. territory.

Another spillover effect that is not directly related to the movement of drugs, guns, or profit is the existence of narco-refugees, or those who have unwillingly left Mexico for the United States due to fear of cartel violence. The existence of these people is an implication of cartel corporate logic applied in Mexico against state agents and innocent citizens. As mentioned in chapter 1, the number of narco-refugees has been rising. Some Mexican analysts have estimated that as many as 200,000 people may have fled just Ciudad Juarez for other parts of Mexico or the United States.[62] Of that number, according to the Ciudad Juarez Citizens Security and Coexistence Observatory, about 124,000 people may have sought safe haven in El Paso.[63] These numbers do not reflect the total number of formal asylum claims but likely reflect those who are using B1/B2 visas that allow them to temporarily visit the United States for a specified length of time but who are now using the visas to live temporarily on the U.S. side of the border. These so-called *inversionistas* work in Mexico during the day but come to the United States at night when the violence is at its worst back home.[64] Several mayors from Mexico's northern border states of Tamaulipas, Chihuahua, and Nuevo Leon have moved to the United States, with some taking up residence permanently and others splitting their time between U.S. and Mexican residences.[65] "The advantage for them is that they cross the Rio Bravo (Rio Grande) and they are in their city hall or their home . . . or govern with the telephone in their hand."[66] The publisher of Mexico's most influential newspaper, Alejandro Junco, moved his family from Monterrey, Mexico, to Texas after he was threatened and gunmen paid a visit to his ranch. Other businessmen from cities across Mexico have done the same.[67] Mr. Junco now commutes every week to Mexico from Texas.[68] In fact, he has publicly called himself a "refugee."[69]

Spill-Back Effects on U.S. Interests in Mexico

The United States is not only affected within its borders by the mosaic drug war in Mexico. Due to the number of U.S. interests in Mexico, ranging from political to social to economic, the mosaic cartel war has touched each in one degree or another. The long-standing relationship between both the United States and Mexico was strengthened with NAFTA, but the relationship is more vulnerable to the actions of violent entrepreneurs operating in a hypercompetitive illegal market.

One of the most visible spill-back effects has included corruption and violence directed at U.S. government posts and personnel. In keeping with its reputation for high-level penetration of governmental structures to gain intelligence, the BLO had an informant who used his job as an Interpol agent working at the U.S. embassy in Mexico City to feed classified information about counter-drug operations back to the BLO.[70] Acts of violence have been directed against diplomatic facilities and personnel. In Nuevo Leon, two vehicles with a number of gunmen attempted to enter the U.S. consulate in Monterrey. The same consulate was the target of a drive-by shooting and grenade attack in 2008.[71] The consulate in Nuevo Laredo was also the target of a grenade attack the following year. A brazen attack against U.S. government interests in Mexico occurred in spring 2010 when three people associated with the U.S. consulate in Juarez were gunned down at the same time. Two of the victims were Americans. The first U.S. law enforcement agent killed in Mexico in twenty-five years occurred in early 2011 when ICE agent Jaime Zapata was gunned down by members of Los Zetas while driving on a highway in San Luis Potosi.

Another very visible spill-back effect concerns the safety of Americans in Mexico. Cartels and gangs in Mexico have also killed American citizens who are not linked to the U.S. government. As mentioned in chapter 1, Mexico is the deadliest place for Americans outside of Iraq and Afghanistan. In 2010, five Americans were killed in Ciudad Juarez in six days. According to the U.S. State Department, in the first six months of 2010, forty-seven Americans were killed in Mexico, while in

2009 there were seventy-nine homicides of U.S. citizens and in 2008 there were fifty-six.[72] Those who were killed fall into a number of categories: innocent victims caught in the crossfire of a shootout, those involved in drug trafficking, those who were in the company of Mexican friends and acquaintances who were targets, and those who were victims of street crimes. Violence aimed at American citizens and American diplomatic personnel in Mexico has prompted the U.S. State Department to issue a number of travel advisories to avoid certain areas of Mexico.

As in the United States, some Americans have been lured into committing acts of crime while in Mexico. American tourists have been approached by drug smugglers to take a small package back with them across the border as a way "to pay for what must be an expensive vacation for the family."[73] The numbers of Americans apprehended as "mules" is difficult to find, but anecdotal evidence suggests that such enticements are routine.

U.S. commercial interests in Mexico have also felt the brunt of the mosaic cartel war. The city of Monterrey has been especially hard hit. As mentioned in the previous chapter, Monterrey experienced an acute rise in criminal violence such as extortion, carjacking, kidnapping, and armed robbery due to its geographic position as the side of the triangle that links it with Reynosa. Known as the "Sultan of the North," Monterrey is a wealthy city that is the home of a number of Mexican companies and American subsidiaries. According to the director of Altegrity Risk International, "U.S. companies see Monterrey as high-risk right now."[74] Tourism in the city is down, which has compounded the sluggish economic recovery following the recession. The American chamber of commerce in Mexico surveyed its members countrywide and found that a quarter of them were reconsidering their investments in Mexico as a result of worries over security; 16 percent of them suffered extortion, and 13 percent experienced kidnappings.[75] Several U.S. companies have decided not to invest in Mexico because of the drug violence; among them were Electrolux and Whirlpool.[76] American importers of fresh fruits and vegetables from Mexico have also been faced with losses due to the withdrawal of a number of U.S. food quality inspectors. Many agricultural inspectors have left or have not been sent because of the fear of drug murders in Mexico, creating delays and bottlenecks that have created additional costs for U.S. food importers.[77]

Such effects on U.S. commercial interests should not overshadow the effects on Mexican businesses. The health of the Mexican economy is also tied to U.S. interests and can add to spillover effects. Many small businesses in Mexico are also at the mercy of the violence. They are extorted by cartels and gangs while facing a drop in revenue due to a decrease in tourism revenue.[78] In Ciudad Juarez, more than 2,500 small grocery stores have closed due to extortion or because customers have left the city; the Mexican social security administration believes that 75,000 residents have lost their jobs since 2007.[79] Without receiving relief, business owners may also become part of the exodus to the United States. When key businesses close, customers who depend on their services also begin to move. In Ciudad Mier, Tamaulipas, medical services were affected by cartel violence. Pharmacies were closing, and the medicine reserves in town began to vanish when delivery drivers were unable to safely travel the highway, fearing they would be attacked on their journey.[80] Oil fields and crop land have also been abandoned in some areas out of fear of being in the crossfire of cartels and gangs. In Tamaulipas, it is thought that about 5,000 ranches may have been abandoned in the state, according to the Tamaulipas Regional Ranchers Association, or URGT. "The industry has been losing money and exports of young bulls to the United States have fallen considerably, [the head of URGT] said. Some 200,000 head of cattle were exported in 2009, but exports will only reach about one-third of that level this year."[81] A steep economic decline may create compounding effects. The number of illegal immigrants to the United States who are not searching for safety necessarily but who are searching for employment, may increase. In addition, a poor employment situation may swell the ranks of gangs and cartels, creating even greater disorder.

Corruption of Mexican institutions also undermines U.S. interests. Having a reliable partner in the south to work on issues of immigration, trade, and crime is a requirement for successful bilateral relations. With corruption having penetrated high levels of the Mexican national government, negotiations and exchanges are often greeted with suspicion on the U.S. side. Such suspicion is also returned on the Mexican side, which often sees the United States as being heavy-handed in its dealings on issues that are seen as directly affecting the Mexican people.

Spill-Around Effects Regionally and Globally

The interests of the United States, as a superpower, span the globe. While not all interests are vital to the survival and continuity of the United States as a nation, the United States still sees regional and international stability as undergirding global peace and prosperity that are integral in the achievement of its vital interests. U.S. global interests and cartels' transnational activities inevitably intersect. The mosaic cartel war is the most extreme manifestation of cartel activities, but not all of their activities are targeted in Mexico and the United States.

The capacity to cross national borders creates several advantages for criminal networks. It enables them to supply markets where the profit margins are the largest, operate from and in countries where risks are the least, complicate the tasks of law enforcement agencies that are trying to combat them, commit crimes that cross jurisdictions and therefore increase the complexity, and adapt their behavior to counter or neutralize law enforcement initiatives.[82]

These qualities of typical transnational criminal networks are mirrored by Mexican cartels because they have expanded their influence outside of the country to acquire necessary equipment and expertise as well as seeking to increase their profits by finding new markets. It is estimated that Mexican cartels have a presence in forty-seven countries.[83] These activities bring with them effects in the region that serve to undermine U.S. interests.

A key U.S. interest in the Western Hemisphere is stability. After the Cold War gripped several countries in Central and South America, plunging them into civil wars, criminality has now become a lethal threat to the sustainability of democratic gains and personal security. Until the 1990s, most countries in Central America contained repressive governments with little solid foundation for democratic institutions or practices. "The political institutions are new, democratic legitimacy is problematic, the countries are poor, social problems huge, the military are supposed to be out of domestic roles and missions, and the police are inadequate."[84] Mexican cartels have contributed to state fragility by working in tandem with criminal groups in the region, which, in turn, contribute to the deterioration of the health of a number of states like Guatemala, Honduras, and El Salvador.

Guatemala has been particularly hard hit by rampant crime; it has a murder rate twice that of Mexico. Widespread criminal violence is causing the breakdown of democratic governance and an erosion of the functional capacity of the Guatemalan state.[85] The first reported Mexican cartel influence came from the Sinaloa cartel in the mid-1990s. Sinaloan preeminence lasted for more than a decade, but since 2005, Los Zetas have begun to assert their own claim to the Guatemalan drug trade. "Police in the suburbs of Guatemala City say many farmers who live along the Mexico-Guatemala border have relinquished their land to Los Zetas."[86] The Zetas are moving south in part to extend greater control over their supply network, and in part to find sanctuary at a time when the Mexican government has launched an all-out offensive."[87] In 2010, six Mexicans believed to be Zetas were convicted in Guatemala for killing eleven people in 2008. The previously discussed working relationship between Los Zetas and the Guatemalan Kaibiles has only further eroded the stability of the Guatemalan state.

In El Salvador, Mexican cartels have forged links with the Mara Salvatrucha-13 gang (MS-13), which is destabilizing the state and eroding personal security in ways very similar to what is occurring in Guatemala. MS-13 originally began as a U.S. gang, forged by El Salvadorans who were war refugees in the United States during the 1980s and who were then deported back to El Salvador after the end of the country's civil war. MS-13 is heavily armed with sophisticated automatic weapons and military-grade explosives because of its access to numerous weapons leftover from El Salvador's internal conflict. MS-13 holds a virtual monopoly on weapons in the black market. In El Salvador, gang-related violence has risen to pandemic levels; it is responsible for 60 percent of all murders.[88] MS-13 has killed a number of state agents and has control over several areas of El Salvador while branching out into Guatemala and Honduras. In fact, MS-13 was responsible for the massacre of twenty-eight bus passengers in Honduras in 2004.[89] The Sinaloa cartel recruited many members to help distribute drugs in the United States and to provide muscle in its war against Los Zetas in Mexico. This gave MS-13 an added infusion of cash, access to new illicit markets, more expertise in the use of violence, greater competence in corrupting state officials, and better know-how to launder money. All of this combined to make MS-13 a more lethal challenge to the health of El Salvador.

Some countries in South America are also connected to the activities of the Mexican cartels. The trafficking of cocaine and heroin from Colombia undermines the country's institutions and the U.S. interests in promoting stability, democracy, and human rights in Colombia. Mexican cartels took over important trafficking nodes from Colombian cartels but still work with smaller cartels and with the guerrilla group Fuerzas Armadas Revolucionarias de Colombia (FARC), which now controls a large portion of the cocaine industry in the jungles and mountains of Colombia. The BLO has been known to buy cocaine directly from the FARC.[90] These transactions provide the guerrillas with much needed money to sustain their movement in the face of constant Colombian political and military pressure. In addition, the preferred transit route for cocaine and heroin exports is through Venezuela, and a string of allegations have been made against the government of Hugo Chavez that it colludes with traffickers for a fee.[91]

Mexican cartel and gang affiliates have been involved in killings in Argentina and Peru, and members have been arrested in Italy and Spain.[92] A connection to smuggle drugs to Japan organized between Mexican cartels and the Japanese yakuza was uncovered in late 2010.[93] To gain access to the lucrative west European cocaine market, Colombian and Mexican cartels have been using countries in West Africa as transit points for smuggling shipments.[94]

Perhaps more serious for U.S. national interests in light of its efforts against al Qaeda is the reach of Mexican cartels' drug dealing. Al Qaeda's affiliates in North

Africa have been engaged in schemes that assist in moving cocaine from West Africa through their territory and into Europe in exchange for a fee.[95] Former chief of the DEA's operations division Michael Braun testified before the U.S. Congress that Mexican drug traffickers regularly mingled with al Qaeda members, "developing relationships that will soon evolve from personal to strategic."[96] In a press interview, Braun raised the stakes by saying that "corporate al Qaeda will be able to pick up the phone to call corporate Sinaloa. . . . It's going to bite us in the ass."[97] Such prospects demonstrate the far-flung effects of Mexican cartel activities and their potential to become spillover effects.

Mexican Cartels as Transnational Violent Entrepreneurs

Mexico's cartels are a menacing presence in a number of different countries for a number of different reasons. The spillover, spill-back, and spill-around effects of Mexican cartel activities on U.S. national interests demonstrate the transnational quality of these violent entrepreneurs. The perpetrators, products, and proceeds of the cartels cross a number of borders.[98] Reflecting the essentially business nature of their enterprise, Mexican cartels mimic legitimate transnational corporations by having a home base in one country where risk is low and operate across the national borders in a number of other states for competitive advantage.

As a result of being transnational actors, the effects of cartels' activities as a function of their corporate logic are intertwined and fuel one another. The effects of cartel activities are not isolated. For example, violent acts against associates and relatives in the United States only further deepen the spiral of revenge in Mexico, feeding the process of high-intensity crime while also sustaining spill-back and spill-around effects. The previously mentioned memo from DHS outlining threats against Border Patrol officers was about MS-13, the Salvadoran gang that has an investment in protecting its smuggling activities due to its empowering alliance with the Sinaloa cartel. MS-13 also has a heavy presence in the United States, with one member sentenced to death on federal charges. Furthermore, instability in Central American countries brought about by thickening criminal relationships with Mexican cartels also contributes to the numbers of Guatemalan, Salvadoran, and Honduran immigrants crossing illegally into the United States. With the number of drugs, guns, and people transiting to Mexico from Central and South America, the southern border of the United States virtually begins with Mexico's southern border.

The most expansive cartel is the Sinaloa cartel, with connections spanning nearly every continent. The Sinaloa cartel in particular appears to have the greatest global span of all the Mexican cartels. It has growing supply links in South America, most notably in Argentina and Uruguay, to gain access to needed precursor chemicals for the processing of meth.[99] In order to make up for the loss of portions of Guatemala as a transit hub to Los Zetas, the Sinaloa cartel has reportedly gained a foothold in Costa Rica.[100] And, on the retail end, the Sinaloa cartel was accused of smuggling five hundred kilos of cocaine monthly into Australia, contributing to Australia's surge in cocaine usage.[101] There have also been reports that the Sinaloa cartel has been engaged in efforts to buy heroin and precursor chemicals from Afghanistan with the assistance of Indian and Turkish criminal groups.[102]

While U.S. interests and cartel activities are far-flung, most unsettling are the spillover effects, particularly the increasing willingness of cartels, gangs, and smugglers to confront U.S. citizens, law enforcement, and government employees with direct violence. Direct and violent challenges to U.S. interests in Mexico have come from each of the cartels and its gang affiliates. This is likely to get worse for two reasons. First, as the United States has improved its border security, smugglers are choosing to go through less protected territory like ranches, national parks, and reservations. Residents and law enforcement in these areas are likely to be outmanned and outgunned, leaving smugglers with a calculus that favors the use of force to escape apprehension and to protect drug loads. This accounts for the increased killings on ranches, lakes, and in national parks. Second, as more vacancy chains are created by incarcerating and killing cartel leaders, lower-level foot soldiers and their lieutenants have moved up in the organizations; this younger generation has an approach to the drug trade that "is less rational and profit-minded than that of their elders."[103] They are more likely to be influenced by narco-cultura and reasons of machismo, which tend to have more violent ends that are separate from earning money. This appears to be part of the reason for the killings of the U.S. consular employees in Juarez. Members of Barrio Azteca, a gang affiliate of the Juarez cartel, reportedly killed the employees in retaliation for the alleged mistreatment of gang members by one of the employees when he was a prison guard.[104]

The combination of less-protected routes being utilized by drug traffickers who are less restrained in their use of lethal force means that violence as a spillover effect is likely to become more visible and therefore more troubling. In past years, traffickers opted to ditch drug loads and weapons as they tried to evade law enforcement. "Now what we're seeing is more of an inclination to just to shoot it out with agents," says T. J. Bonner, president of the National Border Patrol Council.[105] With gangs and smugglers more willing to engage law enforcement in shoot-outs, deaths along the border are likely to rise.

In light of the various effects produced by the mosaic cartel war in Mexico, the current strategies being employed by the U.S. and Mexican governments to defeat the cartels require a review. Up to this chapter, most of this book's emphasis has been placed on the nature of the hypercompetitive illegal market, the nature and actions of cartels as violent entrepreneurs, and what this means for U.S. interests. The following chapter marks a slight shift in emphasis by examining responses, current and future, that are based upon the effects of a mosaic cartel war.

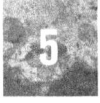

THE "GUARDIANS"
Law Enforcement and the Judiciary

The previous chapters covered the ways violent entrepreneurs in Mexico operate in a hypercompetitive illegal market, leading to a mosaic cartel war and creating the conditions for high-intensity crime. As cartels exercise their corporate logic in the United States, Mexico, and beyond, they affect a variety of U.S. interests. As an extension of one of the central points of this book—that cartels are pursuing profit rather than political change—government is largely seen by cartels as a "third party" in the struggle among rival violent entrepreneurs. "Because there are two groups [a cartel and a rival] fighting for supremacy, anything public servants do that is interpreted as benefiting one group—such as taking down its rival—makes them the target of the other."[1] The U.S. and Mexican governments, through their use of law enforcement and the courts to tackle drug trafficking that can drastically affect profits as well as group autonomy and longevity, are perceived by cartels as a type of "coercive regulating authority." Political leaders, decision makers, law enforcement officials, and military commanders have attempted to reduce the flow of drugs, decrease violence, and reign in public corruption; each threatens the mainstay of cartels and gangs. Dedicated agents of the state see themselves as guardians of public safety and national security, which are threatened by cartels and gangs. State agents generally view themselves as not a third party but a primary party to the conflict. The dedication of the individuals in each government and to the operations to combat the cartels and gangs has varied, especially in Mexico where it grapples with endemic corruption in important state institutions and offices.

This chapter focuses on an important part of the mosaic—government action to combat the cartels. The efforts of the U.S. and Mexican governments are derived from their own corporate logic, or institutional logic. Like their cartel foes, state agents also have pressures and constraints that affect their actions against criminals. These pressures and constraints are acutely felt by democracies that employ law enforcement strategies, operations, and tactics in situations of high-intensity crime. In light of their institutional logic, the U.S. and Mexican governments are attempting to end the mosaic cartel war on terms favorable to them.

Law Enforcement and High-Intensity Crime

For democratic governments like the United States and Mexico, the goal of law enforcement and the judicial system is public safety through the application of laws that are drafted by public representatives accountable to the citizenry. Unlike the unwritten and self-help based laws of violent entrepreneurs' corporate logic, laws governing the institutional logic of law enforcement and the judicial system in democratic nations are enshrined in statutes and enforced by courts. This institutional logic separates high-intensity crime from low-intensity conflict. Counterinsurgency and counterterrorism are not the same as counternarcotics operations (more narrowly) or crime control (more broadly). First, during an insurgency or sustained terrorist campaign, civil rights may be sacrificed in the name of state security. In a police action, civil rights are inviolable. There is a lower threshold for unintentional harm inflicted on citizens, or collateral damage in law enforcement operations and tactics.

Second, the activities that are part of counterinsurgency and counterterrorism operations—target hardening, preemption, resiliency, and recovery—are not typical features of counternarcotics or crime control. Preemption, in particular, can also add to the number of innocent deaths. By striking at threats before they materialize, counterinsurgency and counterterrorism operations will attack potential rather than actual perpetrators of violence. This often leads to the less precise use of force. "Likewise, force used preemptively must be sufficient to overwhelm whatever weaponry insurgents or terrorists might possess. This leads inevitably to an increase in the lethality with which insurgency is met and consequently greater civilian casualties."[2] Due to their links with the judicial system and the need for evidence and warrants, law enforcement participating in counternarcotics and crime control cannot be actively preemptive in their operations. "Preemptive law enforcement" would not only be an oxymoron, but if put into practice, would once again violate a number of civil rights.

Third, the political actors have steered the responses to the situation in Mexico away from those that would be part of the strategies in a low-intensity conflict. In fact, both the U.S. and Mexican governments have been averse to calling the situation in Mexico an insurgency or labeling the cartels as terrorists.[3] While rejecting the labels of insurgency and terrorism when designing strategies to tackle Mexico's high-intensity crime, the United States and Mexico have focused on a judicial and law enforcement approach.

By choosing to rely on a legal framework, certain methods for law enforcement are standard. Michael Kenney outlines the broad institutional logic that police forces in a democracy typically follow: "To be effective, law enforcers must learn how to identify different illegal drugs, initiate investigations against suspected smugglers, gather intelligence from a variety of human and electronic sources, plan and carry out undercover operations, provide persuasive testimony in criminal trials, and conduct a host of related activities, all without violating an assortment of laws and bureaucratic regulations that define acceptable standards of professional behavior."[4] With the power of the state behind it, law enforcement in developed countries generally enjoys an advantage in coercive force that can be brought to bear against criminals. "Armed with sophisticated technologies, professionally trained agents and other accouterments of state power, many law enforcement agencies enjoy a significant advantage in capability over their criminal adversaries."[5] These advantages can be translated into incarceration and seizure of assets that can be used to quell criminal activity.

But law enforcement operations are also at a disadvantage when confronting organized crime because "law enforcers cannot penetrate enterprises they have not identified, nor can they develop intelligence about unknown criminal acts before they are committed. For this reason they usually respond to criminal violations that have already occurred, often between willing accomplices who share a strong interest in shielding their activities from interlopers."[6] Criminals enjoy a "head start" in their activities, which means that law enforcement is playing "catchup" in various ways. "Law enforcers seek to close the gap between their understanding of smuggling methods and what trafficking groups are actually doing."[7] Bridging this distance means that law enforcement must develop surveillance and intelligence capabilities to identify, follow, and deal with criminals while following the law themselves. In addition, after criminals have been apprehended, they must be given an efficient trial and sufficient punishment to not only remove them from operation but to deter others.

However, Mexican governmental agencies have been unable to follow the institutional logic of traditional law enforcement or to use its typical advantages against the cartels. The Calderón administration came into office focusing on job creation, poverty reduction, and crime control. As such, Calderón was putting the Mexican government on a path to bridge the capacity gaps and fill the function holes that have long plagued the state and society. But threatening his three broad goals were

Mexico's endemic corruption sustained by a hypercompetitive illegal market that is flush with violent entrepreneurs. By 2006, Mexican legal structures were at a significant disadvantage and were incapable of effectively engaging in the broad activities of their core functions when faced with the power of the cartels. The larger problem was that law enforcement agencies and judicial institutions were weak and could not close the distance in the "head start" of the cartels; intelligence was often compromised, and cartels enjoyed greater coercive power over police and communities in many areas of the country. This weakness was largely by design of the previous party in power. Under the sustained dominance of the PRI,

> the government of Mexico developed and solidified a centralized structure with an ineffective federal system, an authoritarian political scheme with a strong president, weak and subservient legislative and judicial branches. Such an arrangement allowed the government to cultivate a blueprint of corruption and a lack of accountability by asserting widespread clientelist controls over the Mexican people.[8]

Key to exerting clientelist control was a hollow police force and feeble judicial system. Calderón inherited notoriously corrupt law enforcement agencies at all levels of government, from the federal down to the municipal level. From their inception, the police in Mexico were not designed to be investigative institutions but to provide public order to undergird state stability for the PRI and their various constituents. The police have been generally underpaid, untrained, and underresourced. On average, a Mexican police officer earns about $350 a month, about the same as a construction worker, while not being subject to minimum wage standards or limits on overtime demands as are other public servants in Mexico.[9] Under such conditions, it is no surprise that many officers have been seduced by plata proposals of the cartels. This has led to the poor perception of the police among the Mexican people, 80 percent of whom view the police as corrupt.[10] Further complicating transparency and accountability are jurisdictional issues of the crimes that are perpetrated by violent entrepreneurs—issues that cartels and gangs have been able to exploit. For example, drug trafficking is a federal crime while kidnapping is a local matter.

The judiciary has been similarly hobbled by corruption, low public opinion, complicated procedures, and varying jurisdictions. In a study by the anticorruption group Transparency International, Mexico was ranked among the lowest of over sixty countries in the quality of its judiciary.[11] A report by the United Nations estimated that between 50 and 70 percent of Mexican judges were corrupt.[12] In keeping with the clientelist structure of the state, Mexican citizens have viewed the judiciary as a patronage system, sustained by family ties and wealth. One in three Mexicans admitted to paying a bribe to judges in exchange for a positive verdict.[13] Combined with this toxic mixture was Mexico's unique variation of the inquisitorial system of justice where instead of an instructional judge actively leading the investigation and process of determining a suspect's guilt or innocence, prosecutors were placed in a more central role in the investigation and prosecution of crimes.[14] This subjected prosecutors to inducements and extortion of the cartels.

Tackling "Delinquency" While Taking on the Cartels: Government of Mexico Efforts

In seeking to take on the cartels with the full force of the Mexican government, Calderón in essence tried to disorganize what was already well-organized crime while simultaneously trying to organize Mexico's disorganized institutions to deal with high-intensity crime. Calderón established a security cabinet of over a dozen officials, including the attorney general, secretary of national defense, secretary of the navy, secretary of the interior, secretary of public security, and the director of the Center for Research and National Security (CISEN), which is the national intelligence agency. Under Calderón, the military was deployed to replace or supplement police departments in the most violent areas of Mexico, primarily in cities of the heartland and rimland states. He also launched a series of initiatives to reform Mexican legal institutions and procedures to facilitate prosecutions and incarcerations. It was a wholesale push to give Mexican legal structures the power to follow what is the institutional logic of their counterparts in more developed democracies.

When it has come to addressing the disadvantages and deficiencies of Mexican institutions, Calderón was clear eyed. "To stop delinquency, we first have to get rid of it in our own house," Calderón said in 2008.[15] In the same year, Operacion Limpieza (Operation Clean Sweep or Operation Housecleaning) was launched as part of an effort to root out corruption and inefficiency in the national institutions responsible for tackling organized crime. The operation resulted in the arrests of dozens of officials in the attorney general's office (Procuraduria General de la Republica, or PGR), the office of the secretary of public safety, and the military. Even the former Mexican "drug czar" who served from 1997 to 2000 was arrested for corruption in 2009. The operation also resulted in reforms to improve internal security processes by conducting internal affairs investigations, background investigations, and ethics training and implementing disciplinary actions, as well as measures to improve information security procedures like evidence handling, case file management, and access limitations.[16]

Calderón also created a "disengagement" decree, which allowed for the Mexican government to dismiss any police member without a trial who was believed to be a member of a cartel.[17] In the first eight months of 2010, one-tenth of the federal police force was fired.[18] Pay was also increased to help alleviate the temptation of corruption. Calderón opened a new police academy in Mexico City and beefed up training and recruitment; the numbers of federal officers has risen from 6,000 to 30,000.[19] Another important move by the Calderón administration was to consolidate the two federal police forces (the Federal Preventive Police and the Federal Investigations Agency) into one unit, the Federal Police. It is headed by the nation's top security director, the secretary of public security. This has streamlined federal law enforcement, whereas in the past the two police agencies would be working on the same case without coordinating their actions. Calderón also helped connect the country's disparate police forces in one database to improve intelligence gathering and efficiency, key to closing the head start of criminals.[20]

In tandem with police reform was judicial reform. In June 2008, a major reform to the Mexican constitution was passed, moving Mexico away from its unique variation of the written inquisitorial, confession-based judicial system to an oral adversarial investigations-based system more akin to that of the United States. This transition marked a significant step in making Mexican legal proceedings more transparent and more efficient and ensuring the integrity of the judicial process.[21] The completion of the transition is to happen for all states and the Federal District of Mexico City before 2016, which will then "abandon [Mexico's] centuries-old Napoleonic structure of closed-door, written inquisitions—largely the legacy of Spanish colonial rule . . . the same system that was used during the Spanish Inquisition."[22] Along with constitutional reforms was the establishment of the Special Organized Crime Court, which has jurisdiction over organized crime investigations in the entire country. Having an expansive jurisdiction helps to reduce plata o plomo efforts of intimidation and corruption that were associated with the former requirement that prosecutors go to local judges and courts in cities and towns penetrated by cartels and gangs.

Because these reforms were incipient and the need to quell cartel violence was acute, Calderón embarked on another prong of his strategy. Compensating for the overarching weakness of legal institutions meant turning to the only other part of the state—the Mexican military—that could match the coercive and intelligence advantages of the cartels. Fifty thousand Mexican troops were deployed to various cities where drug violence was the worst, and the hunt began for drug cartel kingpins. "Nearly all large-scale deployments are joint operations with federal police and troops patrolling together, which combines the brute strength of military force with the investigative abilities of the federal police."[23] The government portrayed the use of the military as an interim measure until significant reforms on the civilian side could be instituted and sustained.

The early deployments and actions of the military were focused on the territory of the Gulf cartel and LFM. The Sinaloa cartel began to move against the Gulf cartel in order to fill the gaps left by the Gulf. As a result, violence in Gulf cartel territory rose. The strategy then shifted to a "forest fire" approach—moving into cities where violence was at its worst in an effort to tamp it down. Rather than targeting a particular cartel, the military would respond to the requests of mayors and governors in violent areas. When first assuming their responsibilities in a town, military commanders would vet the local police force for ties to drug crimes. At times, this meant the dismissal of entire police forces. The military has also followed the traditional countercartel strategy of targeting kingpins of the cartels. It has also taken a brute force approach to portions of narco-culture by destroying shrines to Santa Muerte.[24]

Nonetheless, the decision to use military troops was a controversial move. The Mexican military had previously been used only for counternarcotics operations that involved the destruction of marijuana and poppy fields in the countryside. "The army has never worked in urban operations against drug trafficking in urban cells. It's the first time it engaged in urban warfare."[25] In addition, like most standing militaries, troops are not trained for law enforcement. Even though the military is working alongside the police, cooperation has not always been easy. As a result, the use of the Mexican military has proven to be a mixed blessing. Although the drug-related homicides reached their highest level in 2010, jumping by nearly 60 percent from the previous year, the rate stabilized and declined in the last quarter of the year.[26] Violence still grips cities like Juarez and Matamoros, Tamaulipas, and has spread to formerly peaceful cities like Monterrey and Acapulco. The military has been accused of violating human rights and acting outside the law. Several local protests against the military have occurred. The military has also been accused of working for the cartels and gangs in certain areas.

Complicating the efforts of the government have been the differing perspectives that the cartels and the government have when it comes to the geographic dimensions of their respective strategic environments. While the cartels use a geo-criminal lens, the government uses a geopolitical lens. The geo-criminal heartland of the six northern Mexican states does not match the government's geopolitical center in many aspects. The geopolitical center for the national government radiates from Mexico City and comprises most of the states in the cartel rimland and periphery, excluding those in the Baja Peninsula and Yucatan Peninsula.[27] Meanwhile, the states of the geo-criminal heartland have been seen by the national government as peripheral to its geopolitical center. The exception is the city of Monterrey due to its economic, political, and cultural clout. It is the third-largest city after Mexico City and Guadalajara and the financial capital of Mexico.[28] As seen in chapter 3, Monterrey is linked with Reynosa by a highway that is important to Los Zetas and the New Federation for the movement of narcotics to the plazas. Monterrey became a point of convergence for geo-criminality and geopolitics; it is a city that neither the cartels nor the government could afford to lose. But the overall misalignment between what the cartels value as territory and what the government values has created certain gaps in the extension of Mexican government authority. The overall numbers of Mexican police per citizen may be high, but the coverage of certain territory is spotty. Some towns in the northern six states of the geo-criminal heartland have no police at all. The Mexican military and federal police, who have responsibilities aside from battling the cartels, lack the numbers and have not been able to compensate for this shortfall. In addition, historically the states in the geo-criminal heartland have had an uneasy relationship with the central government. This continued during Calderón's time when some governors and mayors of the northern states were from the opposition PRI party and often resented interference from the federal government run by the PAN.

However uneven and embryonic Mexico's approaches have been to address high-intensity crime, the introduction of the military and better coordinated intelligence has caused significant damage to the cartels. "Had Mexico stamped its most-wanted list on a deck of playing cards like the one used in Iraq, the pack would look a lot thinner."[29] Arrests, extraditions, and killings of cartel members all rose under Calderón's leadership. Long resisted by previous presidents, extraditions of drug criminals wanted in the United States increased under Calderón. There were nearly three hundred extraditions between 2007 and 2010. There have been notable successes against cartel leadership. As seen in chapter 2, the BLO has been particularly hard hit by Mexican authorities with the capture of Alfredo Beltrán Leyva in 2008, the killing of Arturo Beltrán Leyva in 2009, the arrest of Carlos Beltrán Leyva in 2009, and the arrest of Edgar Valdez Villarreal in 2010. The Gulf cartel has been stung by a high level loss with the death of its co-leader Antonio Cardenas in 2010. The third in command of the Sinaloa cartel, Ignacio Coronel, was killed in 2010. The leader of LFM, Nazario Moreno Gonzalez, could not escape the reach of Mexican authorities; as mentioned in chapter 2, he was killed in late 2010. Even the leader of the Santa Muerte religion, David Romo, was arrested by authorities in early 2011 for participating in the laundering of ransom money for a drug gang.

Los Zetas have also been damaged by Mexico's efforts. Several cell leaders have been arrested and killed. In addition, other evidence has suggested that Los Zetas's ability to recruit members has been affected by government actions. Many gunmen for Los Zetas who have been captured are less professional than those of previous years; many are teenagers unable to use their weapons or drunks and addicts who are incompetent. Recruitment issues were evident in the attempted move by Los Zetas to press-gang the seventy-two migrants who were then killed for their refusal to work for the cartel. If the numbers for Los Zetas were strong, there would have been little need to force amateurs into their ranks. In some run-ins with the Mexican military, Los Zetas have abandoned the bodies of their fallen comrades, something their group ethos prohibits. This suggests that those killed were also unwilling fighters or that the group ethos of Los Zetas has been weakened.

Prior to the death of LFM's leader, the cartel was offering a truce to the government, perhaps reflecting the government's pressure on the group. The death of LFM's charismatic leader and confusion over his successor was thought to have fatally wounded a once powerful cartel. The Mexican government claimed that LFM had been "completely dismembered," with small splinter groups committing low-level crimes to pay its members.[30] The government's claim was seemingly supported by the cartel itself. Several narcomantas were found in cities in Michoacán and Guerrero that expressed the same sense of finality: "La Familia Michoacana is completely dissolved since it has been unfairly blamed. La Familia Michoacana has exterminated rapists and kidnappers and it's time for Mr. Felipe Calderón to investigate his cabinet, most essentially (Public Safety Secretary) Genaro Garcia Luna."[31] However, with the emergence of LCT as a successor, any optimism must be tempered.

The reduction in violence in Baja California, a state in the heartland of geo-criminality, can also been seen as a success. In less than a year, the state went from being one of the most violent to one of the safest. The change was the result of the arrest of key Tijuana cartel lieutenant Teodoro Garcia Simental, who was responsible for grisly acts of violence; he was responsible for employing El Pozolero, "the Soupmaker," who dissolved bodies of rivals in acid.[32]

Not all of Calderón's efforts were focused on directly attacking cartel and gang members and reforming public institutions. He also took steps to strengthen

Mexican civil society, which was battered by the violence of the cartels. To protect journalists, he created a plan that included "an early warning system in which reporters would have direct access to authorities when threatened, the creation of a council to identify the causes behind attacks . . . and a package of 'best practices' in journalism."[33] In an important test of Calderón's overall strategy, the military's role in Juarez was reduced; many troops were slowly replaced by newly trained federal police in the spring of 2010. In conjunction with a drawdown was the initiation of a campaign called "Todos Somos Juarez" ("We Are All Juarez") that included $270 million to build schools, parks, day-care centers, sports fields, schools, and drug treatment centers and fund hospital renovations, student breakfasts, a youth orchestra, and antiviolence training. Funds were also included to "promote physical fitness, build eco-friendly houses and support free concerts—160 projects in all."[34] However, the security situation in Juarez continued to deteriorate, especially after the car bomb in July 2010. In the fall of 2010, the Mexican military returned to patrol the streets of Juarez.

To Contain and Consolidate: U.S. Efforts against the Cartels

With the escalation of violence in Mexico directly and indirectly affecting U.S. interests, the U.S. government has sought to bolster border security and support the Calderón administration's efforts to break the cartels and strengthen the institutions of the Mexican state. This approach can be labeled as "contain and consolidate"—contain Mexico's violence within that country while helping Mexico consolidate its government reforms to better combat corruption and tackle the cartels. The centerpiece of this approach is the multi-year, billion-dollar Mérida Initiative that was initiated in 2008 by the Bush administration and reauthorized and expanded in 2010 by the Obama administration. In arguing for the passage of the Mérida Initiative in the U.S. Congress, Texas representative Henry Cuellar summed up the thrust of "contain and consolidate": "The levels of violence on both sides of the border now require urgent action on the part of all nations involved. Our own national security is at stake, as are human lives and economic prosperity."[35]

The Mérida Initiative is at its core a joint security plan with four pillars: (1) Disrupting organized criminal groups; (2) institutionalizing the rule of law; (3) building a twenty-first-century border; (4) building strong and resilient communities.

> While the first two pillars largely build upon efforts that began under the George W. Bush administration, pillars three and four broaden the scope of bilateral cooperation under the Mérida Initiative to include efforts to facilitate

'secure flows' of people and goods through the U.S.-Mexico border and to promote social and economic development in violence prone communities.[36]

While the bulk of the Mérida Initiative is focused on Mexico, it also included
assistance to countries in Central America and the Caribbean. The priorities of the
program are strengthening interdiction and enforcement, building institutions,
reducing corrupt practices, and implementing social and economic projects. Yet
the core of the Mérida Initiative was still to provide funding, equipment, and training in support of Calderón's overarching efforts to imbue legal structures with the
institutional logic they were lacking in order to bridge the advantages of the cartels. The funding scheme was clearly slanted in this direction; the overwhelming
proportion of the funding provided equipment and training to Mexican law
enforcement and the military.

The equipment supplied to Mexico was critical in insuring that its institutions
could carry through with its reforms, use the military where needed, and put
Calderón's overall strategy into play against the cartels. Among the equipment was:

- Nonintrusive inspection equipment, ion scanners, and canine units for
  Mexico and Central America to interdict trafficked drugs, arms, cash, and
  persons;
- Technologies to improve and secure communications systems that collect
  criminal information in Mexico;
- Technical advice and training to strengthen the institutions of justice in
  Mexico, including vetting for the new national police force, case
  management software to track investigations through the criminal system,
  new offices of citizen complaints and professional responsibility, and
  witness protection programs; and
- Aircraft to support surveillance and interdiction activities, and rapid
  response of security forces for counternarcotics missions in Mexico.[37]

The Mérida Initiative has also supported Mexico's reforms of its judicial sector.
The United States has helped train judges, police, and military in the United States
as Mexico transitions to an adversarial system of criminal justice. Mexican federal
prisons have also been subject to the wave of reforms. Mexican jails have been manip-
ulated by cartels; the escape of Sinaloa leader El Chapo from Puente Grande Prison
in Jalisco and the prison assassinations his brother and associate in La Palma Prison
are testaments. A new academy to train and vet prison guards was also constructed.

To assist in interdiction of drugs, arms, cash, and people, the United States has also worked with Mexico on more fully securing the border. This includes joint assessments of threats, development of a common understanding of the operating environment, and joint identification of geographic areas of focus for law enforcement operations along with the augmentation of Mexican collection, analysis, and sharing of information from interdictions, investigations, and prosecutions to disrupt criminal flows and enhance public safety.[38] To bolster this array of goals, the United States has helped Mexico establish its own customs and border protection service for the inspection of southbound traffic coming into Mexico.

Community development is a smaller portion of the Mérida Initiative. This portion was designed to sap some of the soft power of the cartels. Secretary of State Clinton explained the reasons for building strong and resilient communities in Mexico: "It's not just security in the most obvious sense, to be safe in your home. It's economic security; it's health security. It's all of the ways that individuals have a chance to lead a productive and successful life. . . . It is about reaching out to and including communities and civil societies and working together to spur economic development."[39] In fact, some of the money for Todos Somos Juarez comes from the Mérida Initiative.

The United States, however, has not relied solely on the Mérida Initiative or the actions of the Mexican government to tackle Mexican cartels. It has taken its own steps within the United States to exploit its more established and less corrupt legal institutions in conjunction with its more sophisticated intelligence-gathering capabilities to contain the more negative aspects of high-intensity crime. There has been enhanced interdepartmental cooperation among the Departments of Defense, State, Homeland Security, Justice, and Treasury and the Office of National Drug Control Policy (ONDCP) to name a few. The level of interagency cooperation among the DEA, FBI, ATF, ICE, CBP, and U.S. Attorney's Offices has also increased.

The Department of State is responsible for coordinating counternarcotics programs implemented by the U.S. government outside the United States. The Department of Defense provides foreign assistance to train and equip foreign militaries for counternarcotics operations; U.S. Northern Command (NorthCom) specifically handles U.S. military interaction with Mexico. Within the United States, the ONDCP is the agency "responsible for coordinating the national drug control effort, promulgating federal drug control strategy, and overseeing the strategy's implementation."[40] However, the ONDCP is not a law enforcement agency. The Department of Justice (DOJ) is the chief federal law enforcement agency that tackles drug cartels and gangs. Within the DOJ, the DEA, FBI, ATF, the National Drug Intelligence Center, the Organized Crime Drug Enforcement Task Force, and the El Paso Intelligence Center all play varying roles in combating drug traffickers and gangs. The DEA, however, has emerged as the main agency in countercartel strategies and operations. The DHS agencies of ICE and CBP maintain a focus on border issues as they relate to smuggling activities northbound into the United States and southbound into Mexico.

These departments and agencies have been involved in a number of cooperative efforts that demonstrate the institutional logic that they follow. The director of the ONDCP (also known as the drug czar) has the authority to designate High Intensity Drug Trafficking Areas (HIDTAs), which are parts of the United States that are known to be important for the production, manufacturing, importation, or distribution of illegal narcotics. One of the twenty-nine designated HIDTAs, the Southwest Border Region includes portions of California, Arizona, New Mexico, and Texas. "The HIDTA collects and shares intelligence and coordinates task forces composed of federal, state, and local agents that target drug-trafficking operations along the border."[41] The Southwest Border Initiative (SBI) is a multi-agency, federal law enforcement operation along the northern side of the geo-criminal heartland that targets the communication systems of the drug cartels. It uses surveillance and wiretaps to track trafficking groups and their product.[42] SBI has sought to gain better control of the border and force potential traffickers and smugglers to the ports of entry where better screening and tracking resources are located. In 2009, DHS secretary Janet Napolitano initiated the Southwest Border Security Initiative. It focused on cartel violence by redeploying personnel to the border and increasing resources for screening cross-border traffic.[43] The interagency efforts were a means to stanch the flow of drugs, cash, and guns between both countries that helps fuel the mosaic cartel war.

Alongside and within these initiatives and interagency actions are more targeted enforcement operations that targeted cartel resources such as guns and money. The Department of the Treasury also maintains the Office of Foreign Assets Control that enforces economic and trade sanctions against international narcotics traffickers, among others, through a Specially Designated Nationals (SDN) list. Individuals and companies linked to drug trafficking may be placed on this list, meaning that their assets are blocked and U.S. citizens generally prohibited from dealing with them.[44] Several dozen Mexican nationals and companies are on the SDN list. The ATF-led Project Gunrunner in 2006 and 2007 was designed to disrupt the flow of guns from the United States into Mexico. It led to the arrest of nearly 1,400 individuals with 850 convictions.[45] Operation Firewall was designed by ICE to combat bulk cash smuggling across the border. ICE also leads the Border Enforcement Security Task Force that targets weapons, narcotics, bulk case, and human smuggling. The ATF gun-tracking operations have not been without scandal. Operation Fast and Furious permitted 1,400 weapons to travel into Mexico that were then subsequently used in homicides; two weapons were used in the killing of Border Patrol agent Randall Terry.[46]

The Department of Defense has also participated in confronting the cartels, mainly by providing assets such as National Guard forces to states that have requested them for border security and by working more closely with the Mexican military than in the years prior to 2006. Operation Jump Start that lasted between 2006 and 2008 put nearly 6,000 National Guard members on the border to support DHS, with Border Patrol being the lead agency. The Guard members did not have law enforcement powers, but the operation was designed to put Guard members in certain roles that would allow more Border Patrol agents to be assigned to the border. In 2010, President Obama authorized 1,200 Guard members from the four U.S. border states to assist DHS in counternarcotics missions on the border. The Guard provided criminal investigation analysts and entry identification teams in support of CBP. The Pentagon has also provided training to the Mexican military in subjects such as planning military operations, using intelligence to find traffickers, and observing human rights.[47] NorthCom has called the new relationship "priority number one," and the Mexican Army has stationed a permanent liaison officer at NorthCom.[48] The command has become a type of clearing house on the U.S. side, helping the various U.S. agencies work together to provide real-time information to those who need it.

Cooperative Institutional Logic: From Mutual Suspicion to Shared Responsibility?

Prior to Calderón's declaration of war against the cartels, the U.S. government was largely focused on strengthening border security and immigration enforcement in the wake of 9/11. Some of the key pieces were:

- Tightening of terrorism laws and expansion of investigative authorities to reduce the risk in the immigrant and non-immigrant admissions process;
- Toughening of the visa, admission, and travel screening procedures at consulates, airports, and ports of entry; and

■ Reinforcing of border security through the expansion of the Border Patrol, especially at the southern border with Mexico, and by the Coast Guard in maritime channels.[49]

The escalation in border security has "translated into tougher laws, rising budgets, and agency growth, the deployment of more sophisticated equipment and surveillance technologies, and a growing fusion between law enforcement and national security institutions and missions."[50] The border evolved into a nexus between public safety and national security, but understanding or accepting this nexus has not been universal. In his book, *The Three US-Mexico Border Wars*, Tony Payan warns against conflating the war against illegal immigration with the war on drugs and the war on terror. "Each problem has its own dynamics, its own actors, its own motives, its own scenarios—even when there are points of intersection among them. Bluntly put, they are not the same issue and they should not be treated as such."[51] While they are not the same issue, the mosaic cartel war inside Mexico has contributed to the fusion of many aspects of these issues. High-intensity crime in Mexico has claimed the lives of thousands of Mexicans; cartels are also involved in human trafficking and smuggling; and cartels take advantage of U.S. immigration law to commit violence in the United States and Mexico.

The actions of the Mexican and U.S. governments show how drug trafficking and cartel violence are reinforcing the interrelationship between many of the issues that define the border. The increased cooperation between the United States and Mexico further demonstrates how both governments are following their institutional logic to play to their advantages against the cartels. An American official summed up the institutional logic that has led to the growing cooperation between the two countries: "The idea is to take our full technological and human capabilities and put them at the service of a willing partner [Mexico] to address what is a crisis situation."[52] To be sure, both sides have had to overcome suspicions and latent animosities. The Mexican government, particularly the army, still resents American seizure of Mexican territory in the nineteenth century while many U.S. law enforcement agencies have been reluctant to share intelligence with their Mexican counterparts out of fear of corruption or incompetence. To thicken these ties and to increase trust between the two governments, the Mérida Initiative Bilateral Implementation Office opened August 2010 in Mexico City as a permanent mechanism for consultation that facilitates the implementation of the mandate of the Mérida Initiative.[53] With U.S. law enforcement and intelligence analysts embedded with Mexican law enforcement units, much, but not all, of the mutual circumspection has been reduced in order to empower institutional logic in the clash against the cartels' corporate logic.

Yet the institutional logic of law enforcement, when clashing with the corporate logic of the cartels, also serves to reinforce it, thereby nurturing and sustaining high-intensity crime. The Mérida Initiative and Calderón's efforts injected greater uncertainty into the hypercompetitive illegal market. Like legitimate entrepreneurs in the licit world, drug cartels seek certainty to create strategies to accumulate profit. However, as violent entrepreneurs, cartels adhering to the dictates of their corporate logic use force and corruption to create some measure of certainty in an unregulated market. Paradoxically, the use of violence and corruption can lead to more uncertainty because cartels and gangs become unsure of their ability to maintain market share in the face of rival cartels or to maintain group cohesion in light of potential traitors. The consequent increase in violence often leads citizens, politicians, and state agents to think that their strategies are unsuccessful.

There has long been a problem of metrics in assessing the effects of law enforcement on drug trafficking. "Any outcome (for example, either a decrease or increase in arrests and seizures) can be politically interpreted as a sign of law enforcement progress and as a sign that more enforcement is needed."[54] Kenney is once again useful to further illustrate the problem: "When drug seizures increase, law enforcers can claim that they are doing a better job of stopping the flow of drugs, or that drug trafficking is increasing, or both—all of which can be used to justify additional funding. At the same time, when drug seizures are down, officials can argue that this is a sign that their efforts are working because smuggling patterns have shifted in response to their activities."[55] The problem is only compounded in a situation of high-intensity crime and a mosaic cartel war where there is an additional metric of assessing the levels and scope of violence as a way to evaluate government success or failure.

Linking common metrics of counternarcotics operations with the desire to reduce violence by destroying cartels through a kingpin strategy is further complicating. It is often unclear if law enforcement strategies to interdict drug shipments and to target cartel leaders are disrupting the cartels in ways that will lead to their dismantling and thereby reduce the levels of violence. For example, in early 2011, the Mexican government secretary, defense secretary, navy secretary, public safety secretary, and attorney general's office said in a joint statement that operations launched by the government in 2010 made significant inroads against the cartels. The statement used drug seizures as a metric. Government operations for the year resulted in the seizure of 11.05 tons of poppy seeds, 21.8 tons of methamphetamine, and nearly 61 million psychotropic drug tablets, more than were seized during any other administration.[56] But the raw number of narcotics seized does not necessarily mean that the cartels' profits are being affected or that this has led to the weakening of the cartels. Without knowing the necessary profit margin of the cartels, such seizures could mean that the cartels are merely producing more narcotics. Ironically, such seizures may also add to the violence, as the person responsible for losing a particular load along with, possibly, the person in charge of the plaza or the particular route will have to answer to someone who paid for its secured delivery. Therefore, violence might be seen as a sign of government success. Intracartel violence can be the result of a successful kingpin strategy. Likewise, intercartel battles can be the outgrowth of government actions to weaken a particular cartel in a given area. In fact, the damage inflicted on the cartels has not translated into the overall lessening of violence or declining of lawlessness in Mexico. Even in some areas of the country where the Mexican government has made large drug seizures or significant arrests, acts of violence have increased along with their intensity. To paraphrase a title of an *Economist* article, rising drug seizures and falling kingpins do not necessarily mean falling violence.[57]

With metrics being interpreted as meaning operations against the cartels could be working or not working, law enforcement and the government also struggle with their own uncertainty. Because state agents may believe that their efforts against the cartels are failing or succeeding (and will seek more funding for resources and greater leeway in either case), cartels resort to strategies that call for more violence and more corruption to counter the moves of the government. "Policymakers are thus confronted with the uncomfortable possibility that increased law enforcement (which leads to increased difficulty and costs to control production zones and smuggling routes, and which in turn leads to the need resolve disputes over territories) could result in increased drug trafficking–related violence."[58] In essence, a cycle not only begins, but perpetuates itself. In many respects, uncertainty on the part of cartels and on the part of the government is the mortar that holds the mosaic pieces in place.

The use of intelligence by governments can never fully eliminate the uncertainty over the use of law enforcement strategies; it can only slightly mitigate it. This need for more information is what has driven greater law enforcement and military cooperation between the United States and Mexico when it comes to the sharing of intelligence. So much so, that one U.S. Border Patrol agent argued that "we need to erase the border on intel."[59] Nonetheless, even if intelligence could be absolutely certain about the efficacy of government actions, law enforcement would still likely seek additional means to either push for a conclusion (if efforts are succeeding) or to alter strategies (if efforts are faltering).

Should the cycle endure or if violence in Mexico intensifies, U.S. interests will continue to be threatened, including its national security. If Mexico continues to suffer the same levels and scope of high-intensity crime, it will be a hobbled partner for the United States when it comes to addressing other common interests that the two nations share. If the violence worsens, the health of the Mexican state may be jeopardized in unanticipated ways. The next chapter will explore a number of scenarios or outcomes of high-intensity crime in Mexico that can help the U.S. and Mexican governments build more successful policies and strategies based on their institutional logic to a degree that can overwhelm the corporate logic of the cartels.

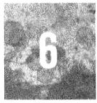

THE HARBINGERS
Possible Outcomes

The main argument of this book is that Mexico is suffering from high-intensity crime and not low-intensity conflict because the main perpetrators are violent entrepreneurs and not insurgents, terrorists, or some amalgam such as "narco-terrorists" or "criminal insurgents." Violent entrepreneurs in the form of drug cartels are following their corporate logic to pursue profit and power in a hypercompetitive illegal market that has been stimulated by the U.S. demand for drugs and allowed to prosper because of Mexico's weak governmental institutions and economic underdevelopment. This dynamic creates value in possessing certain territory for the cartels—geo-criminality—which explains the reasons why violence has occurred in many locations in Mexico but has not engulfed the entire nation. The responses to cartel violence by the U.S. and Mexican governments have been in keeping with the institutional logic of law enforcement and judicial approaches to reduce high-intensity crime rather than the logic of counterinsurgency and counterterrorism, which deal with low-intensity conflict. Nonetheless, the cycle of violence has continued; the mosaic cartel war has become stalemated, and U.S. national security interests remain in peril.

To reduce high-intensity crime, it is essential to examine the directions that the mosaic cartel war might take in the near future. Doing so will allow effective policies and strategies to be developed to prevent or mitigate the worst of the potential effects. Because high-intensity crime better explains the situation in Mexico, the possible outcomes discussed in this chapter bear little resemblance to those that would be associated with insurgency and terrorism. Where there are any similarities they are at the tactical level where cartels and gangs employ coercive and deadly force and where law enforcement attempts to thwart them. Tactical similarities, however, should not be confused with strategic congruence. Sun Tzu is believed to have said that "tactics without strategy is just noise before defeat."[1] Focusing solely on the tactical level without a strategic level analysis invites an outcome of which Sun Tzu apocryphally warned. Therefore, the possible outcomes, or scenarios, described in this chapter focus on the larger strategic level where politics, power, and interests meet. These strategic level outcomes take into account the unique features that contribute to Mexican high-intensity crime such as Mexican politics, society, and economics and how these features interact with Mexico's close geographical relationship with its northern neighbor.

The future of Mexico is not inevitably bleak. Even though death, fear, and corruption continue to occur in many parts of Mexico, aspects that are generally associated with low-intensity conflict are lacking in Mexico's experience of high-intensity crime. However, there are other aspects that do not bode well for bringing high-intensity crime under control in the near future. Outlining what is and is not part of the violence in Mexico provides the parameters of some unique outcomes.

Aspects Not Part of Mexico's Violence

Because many observers have compared Mexico's violence to low-intensity conflict, any parameters of potential outcomes in Mexico must consider aspects that are generally associated with insurgency or terrorism. However, it is clear that several aspects that form the basis for low-intensity conflict are not present in Mexico's mosaic cartel war. If these elements were present, the potential outcomes in Mexico would have different contours and forms. As a mosaic cartel war, the following aspects do not shape the conditions and nature of violence occurring in Mexico.

The Violence Is Not Based on Ethnicity

Unlike many low-intensity conflicts in the post–Cold War era, Mexico's high-intensity crime is not the result of ethnic grievances. The cartels are not an outgrowth of an ethnically based insurgency that has transformed or devolved into organized crime, as occurred in the Balkans in the 1990s. Simply put, the cartels in Mexico are not composed of ethnic minority groups that can portray government actions against them as the product of prejudice or bias. If they were, such claims would elicit a degree of sympathy from outside observers and could possibly lead to increased support from related ethnic communities within Mexico and diaspora communities abroad. If they were ethnically based, law enforcement and the judiciary may have become overly cautious in their operations to blunt any potential for criticism.

The Violence Is Not Linked to Proximity to a Primary Commodity
Unlike low-intensity conflict, Mexico's violence is not about access to a primary commodity. Territory that contains oil, minerals, or even illegal narcotics is not the main point of contention for Mexico's cartels. As seen in the previous chapters, the main source of conflict is access to areas where drugs transit to retail markets in the United States and parts of Mexico. With coca crops located in Colombia, marijuana and opium crops located in multiple rural areas, and meth labs dotting a number of locations, cartels have focused their violence on staging areas, key ports, and critical roadways. The violence has been directed over access to trafficking infrastructure rather than to the commodity at the production level. In fact, the rate at which low-intensity conflicts occur is much higher among drug-producing countries than nonproducing ones.[2] Conflicts that include proximity to a primary commodity have been notoriously protracted. Armed conflicts present many participants with opportunities to exploit commercial resources to pay for military operations and to gain private profit.[3] This linkage contributes to the prolongation of certain conflicts because there is little economic incentive for a warring group to relinquish the profits they receive from illegal trade. Although the violence in Mexico may be prolonged, it is not the result of a dispute over a primary commodity; this dynamic is missing from Mexico's high-intensity crime.

Religion Plays a Minor Role in the Violence and Is Not Its Main Driver
As seen in chapter 2, the narco-cultura of the cartels and gangs is composed of contrived narco-saints and has a linkage with the Santa Muerte tradition. However, this religious symbolism is not a point of contention for the violence in Mexico. The symbols are only a means to provide some legitimacy for the actions of drug traffickers and their enforcers. LFM's and LCT's use of religion was not created to challenge other religious faiths or traditions but to empower their members with the belief that God can serve their interests if they demonstrate their faithfulness in acts of loyalty to the cartel. LFM and LCT have not directly sought to undermine the dominant religions of Mexico. The Mexican government had authorized the destruction of some Santa Muerte shrines, but it was not a large-scale campaign. With 89 percent of the population being professed Catholics, Mexico is one of the top five most populous Catholic countries in the world.[4] The Archdiocese of Mexico has been outspoken against cartel violence and critical of the government response. However, it has also taken a stand against narco-saints and explicitly said that they do not reflect the Catholic pantheon of saints. In short, Mexican high-intensity crime is not a clash of religious creeds that is often part of low-intensity conflicts.

No Significant, Active Insurgent Groups Exist in Mexico or in Neighboring Countries

The lack of insurgent groups in Mexico or in the neighboring countries to its south provides the Mexican state with one less complicating factor. Insurgent groups often have a multifaceted and dynamic relationship with criminal groups. For example, criminals are often recruited to join insurgent movements; some criminals are politicized in jails where many inmates are arrested for participating in violent underground movements. Many insurgent groups also use contacts in the illicit world for funds and supplies. In some cases, insurgents will co-opt the criminal group or attempt to eliminate it because it represents a threat to an insurgent group's authority within a community. In some countries, like Afghanistan and Colombia, insurgent groups and criminal groups can be mutually reinforcing, making it difficult to separate the violence and bring it to a successful conclusion. Although Mexican drug cartels are transnational in their operations and draw on the support of other nonstate armed groups, the support is transactional in nature rather than ideological in affinity. Support will continue as long as financial benefits can be accrued on either side, but any disruption in the flow of money or arms can also disrupt the strength of the relationship.

Governments in Neighboring Nations Are Not Predatory

The Mexican government also has the benefit of neighboring states whose governments are supportive of its goal to defeat the cartels and disrupt the drug trade. No government in the region is actively supporting the cartels. Any cross-border sanctuaries of the cartels are not state-supported and are in fact challenged by neighboring states where cartels are known to have a presence. While corruption is also a problem with states in Central America, these governments are also tackling their criminal gangs and those from Mexico rather than empowering them through direct support. Calibrating policies among governments therefore becomes easier rather than having to contend with a hostile state that would be unwilling to cooperate and even seek to undermine any anti-cartel strategy.

Police and Judicial Reforms Are Not Politicized

The police and judicial reforms put into place by Calderón were not built to serve his particular political faction. The goal was to make the police and judiciary impartial in the enforcement of laws, and they were not reformed as a way to reinforce the PAN's political power by investigating, detaining, and incarcerating its political rivals. This has allowed for a degree of political consensus to emerge over the direction of the reforms that have a better chance of producing a noncorrupt police force and courts. Without a degree of consensus, reforms could have been stymied, giving a distinct advantage to the cartels. The reforms were also not put into place in order to serve a powerful elite, such as the business community, as a means to suppress civil society.

In addition, U.S. assistance, in the form of the Mérida Initiative, follows a good track record of other programs in other countries that have supported police reform. The impact of foreign assistance on reforming police practices has been more likely to succeed when they have supported initiatives that have already been planned or started by foreign governments rather than those that force police to move in new directions.[5]

Mexico's Capital Is Not a Hotly Contested Zone between the Parties . . . at the Moment

Large-scale violence that has gripped other parts of Mexico has not been a feature of the criminal activity in Mexico City. In fact, Mexico City's homicide rate is on par with that of Los Angeles and less than a third of the rate in Washington, D.C.[6] As discussed in chapter 3, Mexico City is far from the geo-criminal heartland under contest by the cartels and has enough distance from portions of the rimland that have experienced violence. Having a peaceful capital allows national leaders the opportunity to meet and deliberate without the additional concern over their personal safety. The administrative capacity of a state is located in its capital. The lack of a stable capital region would be symptomatic of the potential collapse of the Mexican state itself. However, as discussed later in this chapter, the relative calm of the capital could change, further complicating the overall security situation in the country.

Aspects That Complicate High-Intensity Crime

Although there are several aspects that are generally associated with low-intensity conflicts, which are not part of Mexico's high-intensity crime, the situation in Mexico still contains a number of aspects that complicate efforts to bring violence under control. In many ways, this makes the context of Mexico's high-intensity crime more complex than low-intensity conflict.

Mexico Is a Hybrid Node

At the macro-level of international drug trafficking, Mexico is in a unique geographic position that creates micro-level complications for the U.S. and Mexican governments. As previously mentioned, Mexico is a hybrid node, that is, a combination of a source, transit, and demand country. It is also a country that is critical to the northbound trafficking of all the main types illicit narcotics—marijuana, cocaine, heroin, and amphetamine-type stimulants like meth. No other country is a hybrid node or a major depot for the main types of illicit drugs that are in demand. This unique quality makes designing policies and strategies very difficult. First, there is no other similar case from which to draw lessons. The lack of a previous case of success creates additional gaps for policymakers to fill when constructing ways to move forward. Colombia is often looked at as an analogy for Mexico, but Colombia's experience is not the same as Mexico's. The worst period of Colombia's drug cartel violence was in the 1980s, during the Cold War, which served as an ideological prism for understanding cartel violence in the country. The Colombian state was heavily compromised by fighting leftist insurgent groups who were often seen as more threatening to the survival of the Colombian state than the traffickers. Colombia is a source country for cocaine and heroin. The Colombian cartel wars must also be viewed in this context. Although the reasons for the war between the Medellin and Cali cartels are still hotly debated, one possibility is the refusal of Cali to submit to a "supercartel" headed by Pablo Escobar. The Medellin sought, in effect, to be a monopoly over the supply end of the trafficking chain. Another possible reason for the outbreak of Colombia's cartel war of the 1980s is the Cali cartel's decision to shift their distribution through Mexico and lower their transport costs, undercutting the price of Medellin cocaine.

Second, where should governments focus their attention when it comes to Mexico's macro-level position—should they treat Mexico as a source, transit, or demand country? Should counternarcotics strategies be designed along one or more of these features? It is estimated that 30 percent of Mexico's arable land is used for the cultivation of drug crops, with the majority being used to grow marijuana.[7] This means that significant agricultural reforms will be needed in these areas that have had their local economies distorted by drug cultivation.

Third, as a major depot for all the main demand drugs, it is unclear whether successes in countering one drug will have effects on the others. For example, interdiction strategies aimed at marijuana do not necessarily translate into success against cocaine trafficking. A cartel may choose to shift more of its emphasis into trafficking cocaine, which would likely interfere with another cartel's business and set off another round of violence over market share. Finally, the geo-criminality of Mexico also creates difficulties for policymakers; it is not clear if efforts would be best directed in the heartland, rimland, periphery, or some combination. The Mexican government may become more interested in reinforcing peaceful and important parts of the geo-political core.

Mexico Is a Fragile Democracy

Mexico's democracy is less than a hundred years old and was characterized by one-party rule for a majority of the years after the Mexican Revolution. Although institutions of the Mexican state mimicked democratic practices, they were hollow and did not reinforce principles, like the rule of law, that are critical to a democratic republic's durability. This makes the sustainability of Calderón's reforms aimed at strengthening the pillars of Mexico's democracy an open question. The weakness of Mexican democracy may undermine any positive growth in the institutional logic of the judiciary and among law enforcement.

Very troubling are public perceptions of democratic practices among the Mexican people. Public support for democracy in Mexico is low. In a recent poll by Latinobarometro, less than half of Mexicans believe that democracy works in their country—the lowest score among the eighteen countries surveyed.[8] In a 2010 poll conducted by the Mexican newspaper *El Milenio* found that 59 percent of Mexicans believed that the cartels were winning the drug war, while only 21 percent believed the government was winning.[9] Such a weak belief in the efficacy of their democracy among Mexicans suggests that institutional reforms may be easily stymied by a civil society that can be more easily influenced by cartels and their mix of soft power and coercion. A report by the UN Office on Drugs and Crime found that people in fragile democracies "often interpret rising crime rates as evidence that constitutional protections have been extended too far."[10] This can lead the public to demand the government reduce civil rights guarantees.

Mexico Has Continued to Rely on the Military for Law Enforcement

The use of the Mexican military to bolster law enforcement efforts has brought some success in removing many cartel leaders from positions of power. However, the long-term use of the military in counternarcotics roles has led to many drawbacks. The use of such a strategy has tempted and personally enticed many members of the military who are involved in counternarcotics operations. The lucrative nature of drug trafficking has corrupted many military commanders who saw opportunities for personal enrichment. Corruption of the Mexican military has already surfaced. A number of soldiers have been arrested for accepting payments from a drug cartel to provide intelligence about government operations against drug gangs.[11] The use of the military in other countries for counternarcotics operations has crippled the effectiveness of not just the counternarcotics strategy but also the core war-fighting competencies of the military.

In addition, human rights concerns have typically arisen in other instances of military actions in the realm of law enforcement. Soldiers are not trained for key interactions with the public when it comes to dealing with crimes. In Mexico, there have been charges by the public that the military has engaged in torture and disappearances.[12] Mexico's National Human Rights Commission has logged a large increase in the number of abuse claims against the National Defense Ministry since 2006.[13] The UN has also called on the government to remove the military from policing duties.[14] Human rights concerns can also be used by the cartels to generate popular opposition that leads to political pressure to remove the armed forces from the streets, allowing a freer hand for the cartels. Human rights concerns may also affect U.S. funding for the Mérida Initiative. Releasing funds for any efforts to tackle drug cartels will face obstacles from members of the U.S. Congress who believe that foreign aid to police agencies and militaries must be linked to the upholding of basic human rights in those countries. When these concerns are combined with U.S. budget concerns, the overall effect may be to reduce or eliminate Mérida Initiative support, leaving Mexico to fend for itself.

Traditional "Post-Conflict" Inducements Are Inappropriate

Paths out of low-intensity conflicts for irregular fighters are not ones that can be offered to drug cartels in high-intensity crime. As discussed in chapter 1, brokering agreements with violent entrepreneurs to surrender is illogical. Disarmament, demobilization, and reintegration (DDR) schemes used to induce insurgents into legitimate politics are wholly inappropriate in the case of drug cartels. For example, it is highly unlikely that the Mexican government would offer positions in the police force or military to gang members or cartel enforcers who renounce violence and stop dealing drugs. It is also equally unlikely that a cartel leader such as Joaquin Guzman would relinquish his position as the head of the Sinaloa cartel in exchange for a position in the political arena of Mexico if offered the opportunity.

A voluntary reduction in violence by the cartels in exchange for government amnesties or pardons would be difficult for cartels and gangs to undertake. As seen in chapter 2, the corporate logic of cartels requires them to use a certain level of violence. In fact, it is their ability to wield violence successfully that allows them to thrive in a completely unregulated market. Even if cartels and gangs renounced drug trafficking, the individual skills and abilities of their members mean that they can employ them in other black market enterprises such as smuggling and trafficking human beings, counterfeit consumer goods, vehicles and parts, and whatever seeks to illegally cross the U.S.-Mexico border and can make a profit.

Again, unlike insurgency or terrorism, "organized crime has always prospered where international boundaries meet, but any nation whose standard of living is higher than its neighbor must recognize this threat. . . . One has a natural incubator in which transnational organized crime can grow and prosper."[15] The abiding inducements to enter and continue criminal enterprises make the cessation of organized crime—and the violence that comes along with it—complications that Mexico and the United States may never be able to fully bring under control.

Mexico: Two Ends of the Spectrum

There are a number of possible scenarios for the direction of Mexico's bout with high-intensity crime. Based on this book's thesis, the following scenarios do not mirror scenarios that would be traditionally associated with low-intensity conflict because many of its aspects are not part of Mexico's violence. The aspects that are part of the violence create the contours for a number of directions that Mexico's possible future might take; these scenarios exist within a spectrum, ranging from the defeat of the cartels and the success of U.S. and Mexican government efforts on one side to the collapse of the Mexican state on the other.

On one side of the spectrum is a possible scenario where the Mexican state, with continuing assistance from the United States, prevails against the cartels, and the scope and levels of violence are lowered. Such an outcome would "build from the strength of Mexican civil society, cultural institutions, and efforts toward reinforcing a stable democracy."[16] Better integration of intelligence and improved coordination among law enforcement and the military, along with more efficient courts, would succeed in dismantling the major cartels and suppressing drug trafficking. In tandem with state actions would be the active resistance by civil society to drug crimes and the growth in links between the state and local communities. Community programs and development projects in areas where drug traffickers recruit young people would successfully steer them toward legitimate employment. In effect, the Mexican government reforms take hold, and citizens begin to embrace the new strength of state institutions.

Also, the Mexican state might benefit from a significant alteration or disruption in the hypercompetitive market for illegal drugs such as Colombian cartels returning to Caribbean smuggling routes for cocaine, cutting out Mexican cartels as middlemen. Drug trafficking and its related crimes return to being a manageable law enforcement issue, with the military returning to its traditional role and responsibilities. In essence, the Mexican state emerges as a type of market enforcer in the hypercompetitive illegal market by reducing the power of violent entrepreneurs to exert their corporate logic. Another disruption may be a drastic reduction in U.S. demand for illicit narcotics. This may be achieved through better law enforcement or a new paradigm shift such as drug legalization.

Should the Mexican state prevail, the benefits to the United States would be dramatic. Spillover, spill-back, and spill-around effects would be reduced. Notably, drug crimes in the United States related to Mexican high-intensity crime would decrease. Border security would focus more intently on other important issues like human smuggling and trafficking as well as preventing potential terrorists and dangerous materials from entering U.S. territory.

This scenario is highly unlikely to occur in the short-term while the long-term prospects are also bleak. The key reason is Mexico's location and the consequent geo-criminality that it produces. Unless there is a drastic alteration or disruption in the patterns of regional drug trafficking, the United States and Mexico will have to figure out the right strategic equation to tackle the macro-level drug trafficking aspects of Mexico's place as a hybrid node and major depot. A change in routes by Colombians would still leave the markets for marijuana, Mexican tar heroin, and meth untouched. A significant disruption may also create the conditions for more violence as the effects on profits may lead to internal splits within cartels and gangs and make competition over shrinking spoils among cartels and gangs more acute. The lucrative nature of the drug trade means that cartels can outspend the government where it needs to—bribing state officials and law enforcement, recruiting new members, and buying more sophisticated weapons and surveillance technology. The arrest of the head of Mexico's Interpol office for corruption demonstrates the extent of plata o plomo. The reforms put in place by Calderón can be easily swept aside by a tsunami of cash or powerful coercive threats.

Additionally, while the Mexican government has adapted itself to combating high-intensity crime, cartels may also evolve to sustain themselves in a hypercompetitive illegal marketplace. Some may become extinct due to a combination of government pressure, internal fragmentation, and aggressive competitors. Some may become smaller cartels, or *cartelitos*; the landscape of Mexican organized crime may come to resemble a "patchwork of dozens upon dozens of baby cartels."[17] Cartelitos may begin to specialize in one drug, be located in a specific portion of the heartland, rimland, or periphery, or perform a specific task such as moving shipments from a port to a plaza.

On the other end of the spectrum is the fear that Mexico collapses and becomes a failed state. With many zones of impunity and with many cities and towns without effective governance, cartels have already "hollowed out the state" to a certain degree. This hollowness means that the Mexican government is unable to control some portions of its territory. According to a Pentagon study that listed Mexico as a state ripe for collapse, "The government, its politicians, police, and judicial infra-structure are all under sustained assault and pressure by criminal gangs and drug cartels. How that internal conflict turns out over the next several years will have a major impact on the stability of the Mexican state. Any descent by Mexico into chaos would demand an American response based on the serious implications for homeland security alone."[18] Mexico may not be on its way to becoming a "narco-state," but there are several "narco-cities" in Mexico. A 2011 report from Mexico's national secretary for public safety reveals that the country is growing slightly more violent, with the violence becoming significantly more dispersed.[19] A number of narco-cities strung together or an increase in their number would lead to an expan-sion of the zones of impunity, weakening the overall health of the Mexican state. State collapse in Mexico would come as zones of impunity expand and violence came to engulf areas of the geo-criminal periphery that overlap with the geo-political core. In this scenario, the best that Calderón's reforms would have produced would be to have merely temporarily damaged the cartels and marginally improved key institutions of the state in unsustainable ways. The worst that Calderón's reforms would have produced would be more cartel violence against the state, civil society, and each other, leading to an unstoppable deterioration of the security situation in the country.

Mexican state failure would likely start with the armed forces coming under increasing strain with large-scale and long deployments; corruption may begin to have a corrosive effect on an institution that is relatively respected by civil society. Security personnel would desert en masse, leaving citizens exposed to the predations of cartels and gangs. Brian Jenkins described the contours of this scenario:

> The deterioration of northern Mexico from crime-ridden to crime-ruled is likely to be gradual and insidious. Nominal state authority would still exist. Police would continue to deal with petty crime. Commerce would continue. Superficially, northern Mexico might appear normal—a failed state does not necessarily have to look like Somalia. But no-go areas and untouchable crime bosses protected by heavily armed private armies would point to the real locus of power. [20]

Civil society would come to be ruled by fear, and the economy would cease to function effectively as more middle class professionals begin to leave the country.

More Mexican narco-refugees would seek asylum in the United States, and spillover and spill-back crime would rise.

Many elements already appear to be in place for the Mexican state to fail; chief among them is Mexico's democratic institutions. Public support for them is relatively low. This does not mean, however, that the state itself is susceptible to collapse; Mexico is not likely to fall into the disorder and anarchy that have gripped other nations such as Somalia, Pakistan, and Yemen. "Mexico still has strong institutions that millions of people work and struggle every day to defend, including relatively well-functioning public services such as health and education. Judicial, political, and military institutions, while far from perfect, can hardly be described as on the verge of collapse."[21] There are several reasons that little will undercut this description. First, there is no significant insurgent challenge that can severely damage the main organs of the state, most notably the military. The armed forces of Mexico still remain loyal to the government, and civilian authorities still maintain authority. Second, Mexico has portions of its territory that are violent, but the nation is not out of control. Most of the violence is located in the geo-criminal heartland, with levels in the state of Chihuahua and its city of Juarez being especially intense. Mexico ranks sixth in the world behind India, Russia, Colombia, South Africa, and even the United States in terms of homicides.[22] Third, and most crucially, there has not been a coup or any extraconstitutional moves against the government or any significant division within the government that would bring about fragmentation of political order that often precedes the collapse of the state. Mexico has not experienced a violent takeover of its government or a coup, unlike nineteen other Latin American nations in the twentieth century. In many respects, "the violence epitomizes the will of the people carried out by a democratically elected government against the cartels."[23] Finally, Mexico's financial system and economy have been resilient in the face of high-intensity crime and the global recession. Mexico has not experienced hyperinflation or a sudden, rapid decline in economic stability. All of these elements point to the relative durability of the Mexican state.

Although Mexico will not become a failed state, neither will it be a strong one. Rather than falling completely on one side of the spectrum or the other, Mexico is likely to struggle somewhere in the middle, between a fully functioning state with a high degree of law and order and a failed one marked by the lack of governance and security in all of its territory. The desire of the Mexican government to tackle the cartels and lower the violence will continue to clash with the incapacity of the Mexican government to make headway. Mexico will be an enfeebled state, battered by drug cartels and dependent upon U.S. assistance. Such a condition will lead to a number of possible outcomes.

Possible Outcomes for Mexico: Between Government Success and State Failure

One possible scenario is the emergence of the "new abnormal," meaning that the current violence will become a regular feature of Mexico. A stalemate between the cartels and the Mexican government will continue. In this scenario, drug violence in Mexico will become "a fact of life" in relations between the United States and Mexico. Drug gang and cartel violence will continue to seep into the United States along with the supply of drugs. Flare-ups in Mexican violence will be followed by periods of calm, only to be followed by the return of familiar patterns of killings and mutilations. Due to the presence of the military in combination with better policing and more incarcerations, homicide rates may stabilize or decline in certain cities but rise sharply in new cities. Outlines of this scenario were becoming visible in late 2011, with Mexico's national secretary of public safety reporting that Juarez and Tijuana were becoming safer while Monterrey and Acapulco were becoming more dangerous.[24] The new abnormal would likely mean a slow but steady number of narco-refugees coming to the United States. Pressures from many quarters of the American public for more adequate responses would be placed on decision makers—on one side would be those seeking more expeditious forms of action for tackling the source of violence in Mexico; another side would likely wish to either continue the policies to assist the Mexican government without direct intervention.

Rather than collapse, the new abnormal depicts a Mexican government that adapts to the forms of violence, as does civil society. For example, during the 2010 holiday season, the Mexican government recommended that Mexicans in the United States who want to travel back to Mexico to visit family should group together with others to move in convoys and only in daylight hours.[25] Once the convoys checked in with Mexican federal authorities, they were escorted and monitored with assistance from the Mexican military. Cartels and gangs would also adapt to the pressures from the effects of the Mérida Initiative. With improvements at ports of entry, cartels would design more inventive circumvention techniques to move drugs across the border. For example, in the years 2008 to 2009, there was a 63 percent increase in the number of tunnels discovered underneath the border.[26] This is a response to more Mexican and U.S. law enforcement operating along the border above ground; the cartels and gangs have simply excavated more tunnels to move drugs (and people) underground.

As the cycle of adaptation continues, cartels and gangs will likely become more violent in their confrontations with U.S. law enforcement as a way to break out of the cycle and deter officials from interdicting loads and detaining members.

There is also the danger of an "accidental narco" syndrome developing in Mexico. Unlike the balloon effect of counternarcotics operations spreading the trafficking of drugs in other regions, and unlike David Kilcullen's notion of the "accidental guerrilla" whereby pursuit of jihadist terror groups only leads to the creation of more, the accidental narco refers to the Mexican government becoming a type of cartel enforcer in its own right. Tempted to show progress to the U.S. and the Mexican people in lowering drug violence, the Mexican government may choose to collude with some of the less violent cartels in order to gain intelligence and information to use against the most violent cartels. In essence, the government becomes an armed wing of the cooperative cartel or cartels by clamping down on rivals and arresting their members. Depending on the scope and intensity of the Mexican state's actions, violence could increase in the near term or become protracted depending on the capabilities and will of the targeted cartels. There has been a glimpse of this with the car bomb detonated in July 2010. As mentioned in chapter 2, the Juarez cartel detonated the bomb in the belief that the Mexican government was siding with its rival, the Sinaloa cartel. Mexican civil society may also become more cynical of the government and the military if they appear to be picking sides with a cartel that is not from the "home team."

Under an accidental narco scenario, a protracted and bloodier campaign may ensue as the cartels and government begin to use violence as a method of deterrence. The United States will be torn between supporting the Mexican government's strategy and criticizing it for not fully combating all the cartels. Cartels may also begin to more actively target U.S. interests if they believe the United States is supporting the Mexican government's targeting of them over their rivals. Faced with what might appear to the targeted cartels as an all-out effort against them, they would be little deterred from using more violent tactics against state agents. The targeted cartels may even band together and form an alliance of convenience to combat the U.S. and Mexican actions.

The formation of such an alliance may also occur under another scenario—"pax narcotica." A balance of power may emerge among the cartels with clear spheres of geo-criminal influence, division of labor, or specialization of skills. One cartel may become the obvious hegemon and serve as a regulator in the hypercompetitive illegal market. The current violence in Mexico may be seen as a consolidation phase; the mosaic cartel war is a process for some cartels or a single cartel to consolidate the various factions and cliques that are bringing inefficiencies to the hypercompetitive illegal narcotics market. For example, the New Federation may prevail against Los Zetas and become a type of "concert of cartels" that acts as a type of board of directors that will manage disputes among the participants in the hypercompetitive illegal marketplace.

After consolidation, a tacit deal may then be cut with the government to permit the cartels to traffic drugs without high-level violence in exchange for limited prosecutions and the end of extraditions to the United States. Two former senior members of PRI and PAN governments have previously suggested such a deal. Former foreign minister Jorge Castaneda suggested illegal activities by the cartels would be permitted if they curbed public violence.[27] President Fox's former spokesperson, Ruben Aguilar, argued that "we must constrain the actions of organized crime, obligate them to obey the rules of operation and in this context, we would have to accept the possibility of . . . legalizing the sale of drugs under certain agreements."[28] In the run-up to the Mexican presidential election in 2012, the PRI was vague in how it would handle drug violence, and its standard bearer for the presidency, Enrique Pena Nieto, was elusive in answering questions about the way forward.[29] One of the PRI's leaders in the senate seemed to pine for a return to the old understandings between it and the cartels by saying that when the PRI was in power, "I never saw a decapitation in the streets of Mexico."[30] As previously mentioned, at least one cartel, LFM, had proposed truces with the government and promised a reduction in violence if the government focuses more on targeting its adversaries. At the end of 2010, LFM sought to disband under certain guarantees from the Mexican government.[31] However, its offshoot, LCT, has not relented in its killing nor has it ended the trafficking of drugs initiated by LFM.

Rather than viewing a government rapprochement with the cartels as the failure of the rule of law, Mexican civil society may become amenable to pax narcotica, making such tacit deals more broadly acceptable. In the latter part of 2010, Mexicans appeared to be experiencing war fatigue; for the first time since Calderón declared war on the cartels, a plurality of Mexicans considered the campaign a failure.[32] Under such a "peace," however, it would be difficult to know where the drug cartels' influence on Mexican politics begins or ends, or even if the government has any means to affect the actions of the cartels should they step outside the tacit agreement. Pax narcotica could be just a step in the direction toward the Mexican state becoming a full-blown narco-state, meaning even more difficulties for the U.S.-Mexican relationship. The U.S. government would likely increase its pressure on Mexico to clean up its corrupt deal-making, while the Mexican government would be at the mercy of the threats of the cartels to return Mexico to high-intensity crime.

Finally, a "Zeta state" might emerge. This does not mean the collapse of the Mexican state and the replacement by Los Zetas. Rather, Los Zetas and other violent actors may evolve (or devolve) into militias alongside the proliferation of private security firms hired by wealthier Mexicans to protect them from drug violence and armed vigilante groups to protect poorer communities. "The traditional tools of the state to enforce law will no longer work, for organized crime has become part of the state; a state within a state."[33] The Mexican government would be in control of its geopolitical core/geo-criminal periphery and "strategic facilities such as major ports, airports, oilfields, refineries, energy generation, food production, and major highway systems."[34] A type of shadow state may emerge, with these groups drawing more and more legitimacy away from the Mexican state, which will be viewed as increasingly powerless to curb lawlessness.

There are already some hazy outlines of this scenario. Many companies, both Mexican and foreign, have hired security firms to patrol their business and track the transportation of their merchandise. Armed vigilante groups have already sprouted up in several Mexican states. The Citizens' Command for Juarez, which is financed by businessmen, promises to "end a criminal's life every twenty-four hours" and considers itself to be the "first citizens' post-revolutionary movement"; the Popular Anti-Drug Army has been hanging banners in various cities in Guerrero and Morelos challenging the cartels; a rancher in Guerrero formed a group called the Army That Liberates the People and has hung banners with messages that threatens the region's drug traffickers as well as praising the Mexican military "for its achievements in the struggle against drug trafficking."[35] As one expert on organized crime states, "The paramilitary model in Mexico is different from Colombia. In Colombia irregular troops are organized to take over territory, houses, etc. In Mexico paramilitary communities are created. They infiltrate them, they prepare them, and then become paramilitary communities."[36]

Such an emergence of a Zeta state may create even higher levels of violence in Mexico as the proliferation of armed groups makes alliances, truces, and ceasefires even more difficult to achieve. The number of people under private arms in Mexico has already ratcheted up killings; it is plausible the adding more people and more weapons may do the same. The response of the Mexican government may be to rein in such groups, potentially sparking more violence. The United States may witness even more spillover violence and more illegal weapons trafficking as groups in Mexico begin to arm themselves in greater numbers.

None of these scenarios are mutually exclusive, nor would each scenario need to apply to the entire country of Mexico. States may find pockets of these conditions with cities and towns being compromised. "Zeta cities" may emerge under the broader conditions of pax narcotica. Pursuit of an accidental narco strategy by the government may lead to a Zeta state, while the new normal could presage the development of pax narcotica. There are a multitude of possibilities; each of the four would mean significant adjustments by the Mexican and U.S. governments and changes in the tone and perhaps nature of the relationship between the two countries.

Warning Signs Ahead?

There are warning signs of a more significant turn for the worse that may lead to the fulfillment of the potential scenarios detailed above. First, if there is a very sharp increase in the proportion of homicides that include agents of the state. As mentioned in the first chapter, less than 10 percent of cartel targets are members of state agents, while chapter 3 identified the areas where the most of their killings have occurred. Especially troubling would be a rise in targets among the military. While several members of police departments have sought safety in the United States, no members of the Mexican military have done so. If there is a noticeable trend in Mexican military members becoming narco-refugees, this means that the most coercive arm of the state does not believe that it can prevail against the cartels nor do its members feel that they are safe from personal reprisals. Similarly, if the Mexican military merely "returns to barracks" and refuses to participate in any future campaigns against the cartels, then this too would be a decidedly negative indication. Ominously, the revenge killings of the family of the Mexican marine who shot and killed one of the leaders of the BLO speaks to the power of the cartels to reach out and inflict pain on select members of the Mexican security apparatus. The open question is whether other cartels could do so on a much wider scale.

Second, an increasing "brain drain" of educated and prosperous Mexicans would also indicate that the security situation continues to be poor or is deteriorating. Currently, the shaking down businesses for "protection" money, kidnapping businessmen and professionals for ransom, and murder-for-hire schemes occur with or without any linkages to the drug trade. These activities act as stand-alone profit-making activities and form the equivalent to "a parallel tax system that threatens the government monopoly on raising tax money."[37] The significant pay received by gangs acts as an incentive that perpetuates the occurrence of violence.[38] In a country with significant disparities in wealth, these activities are likely to be perpetuated, meaning more middle-class Mexicans may decide to leave their country. "One young Mexican executive at cement giant Cemex SAB, which has headquarters in Monterrey, said he can count at least twenty different families from his circle of friends who have left—nearly all of them for nearby Texas."[39]

A brain drain may foretell a third worrying indicator—a sudden economic decline in Mexico related to drug violence. As discussed in chapter 4, there are some haunting indications from the city of Monterrey with the number of U.S. businesses reconsidering their investments and professionals deciding to leave the city. In the estimation of J.P. Morgan's chief economist for Mexico, the country likely lost approximately $4 billion in investments in 2010 when companies reconsidered their plans to invest because of drug violence.[40] In the geo-criminal heartland and the rimland states of Durango, Sinaloa, and Michoacán, foreign investment dropped to roughly $1.9 billion in 2010 from an average of about $5 billion a year from 2005 to 2008.[41] Many businesses in Mexico are also at the mercy of the violence. They are extorted by cartels and gangs while facing a drop in revenue due to a decrease in tourism revenue.[42] Oil fields and cropland have also been abandoned in some areas out of fear of being in the crossfire of cartels and gangs. In the Burgos Basin, the site of Mexico's biggest natural gas field in the state of Tamaulipas, gunmen seized the Gigante Uno gas plant and kidnapped five Pemex workers. According to a recent press release from the Mexican senate, "The unsafe conditions are preventing Pemex from extracting 150 million cubic metres of natural gas in the Burgos Basin."[43] Should this pattern expand, the economic impact on the Mexican economy could become more acute.

A fourth worrying sign would be significant violence aimed at national politicians in Mexico. The trend in assassinations and attempted assassinations is not reassuring. In 2008, eleven men were arrested and accused of planning a high-level assassination with the possible collaboration of Mexico City police and former army soldiers.[44] The bulk of cartel assassinations of governmental figures has been limited to police officers and mayors, but a leading politician who was almost certain to win the governorship of the northern state of Tamaulipas was assassinated just days before the election. He had pledged to be tougher on organized crime than his predecessor. With the kidnapping of former presidential candidate Diego Fernandez de Cevallos, who is a power broker in Calderón's ruling National Action Party (PAN), the possibility of more visible displays of violence directed at higher profile national politicians cannot be discounted. Shockingly, in late 2008, a major in the Mexican army who was part of President Calderón's personal security detail was arrested for being on the take of the Beltrán-Leyva cartel. He is believed to have passed along information regarding the activities and travel plans of the Mexican president.[45]

Finally, another warning sign would be if the capital, Mexico City, becomes a zone of insecurity. The pulse of any nation is its capital. If that heart rate comes to be at the mercy of civil violence, the health of the rest of country is put in jeopardy. Citizens begin to question the very legitimacy, authority, and capacity of the state to meet their most fundamental needs. Mexico City has been plagued with high levels of street crime and police corruption, but as mentioned previously, it has been relatively immune from the types of violence that has gripped border cities in the heartland of geo-criminality. As covered in chapter 3, the capital has been largely a place of peace where high-level drug traffickers coexisted with each other and the government. But with a more confrontational stance taken by the parties, a number of high-level drug cartel members have been arrested or killed near the capital. The sons of Sinaloa and Gulf cartels were caught in the upscale suburbs of Mexico City; Edgar Valdez Villarreal of the Beltrán-Leyva Organization was caught in Morelos near Mexico City; and Arturo Beltrán Leyva was killed in a town in the state of Morelos. Cartel violence has also been slowly inching toward the capital. In 2008 alone, three senior law enforcement officials were assassinated: Roberto Bravo, director of investigations of the Sensitive Investigations Unit of the federal police; Edgar Gomez, general coordinator for regional security at the Mexican secretary of public security; and Igor Calderón of the Federal Investigative Agency. In the same year, the editor of *El Real* newspaper was shot to death as he drove in a Mexico City suburb. In Cuernavaca, four decapitated men were hung from a bridge on August 23, 2010. Cuernavaca is a favorite destination for residents of Mexico City and is just over fifty miles away.

Turning Mexico City into a battleground is not out of the realm of the possible if cartels and their enforcers feel that the government is giving them no choice but to strike deep at the heart of the state's power. If the cartels act against the political and business elites in the capital, they will place greater pressure on the government to act. Another concomitant danger is the rise of more violent cartel and gang lieutenants who are filling the vacuum created by the government's arrests and killings of high-level cartel leaders. These lieutenants are more willing to use violence to settle disputes. Therefore, the tacit links between traffickers and politicians would be disrupted even further, likely leading to the types of violence seen in the heartland states where broken links precipitated the cartel wars of the past and present. In 2011, there were three hundred gangland-related homicides in the Mexico City metropolitan area, an unprecedented number.[46]

Furthermore, if the cartels begin to focus on Mexico City as a larger retail market, this may also stimulate more intercartel rivalries. This may occur if access to the U.S. market becomes constricted to an extent that profits are affected by law enforcement. Mexico City has a population of over 20 million and is larger than any city in the United States, making it an enticing pool of potential customers. Turning it into a more significant retail market may enhance its importance to the overall drug trade in Mexico and the region, thus stimulating the more violent parts of the cartels' corporate logic. And, because of hybrid quality of Mexico's status in drug trafficking, any shift in the market may also redraw the lines of geo-criminality. Mexico City may emerge as a portion of the heartland and, when combined the city's status as the geo-political core of the government, could create the type of violence seen in Monterrey when these critical geographic priorities of the government and cartels overlapped.

A Potential Strategic Shock for the United States

The product of the scenarios might be what Nate Freier terms "strategic shock" whereby

> the unanticipated onset forces the entire defense enterprise to reorient and restructure institutions, employ capabilities in unexpected ways, and confront challenges that are fundamentally different than those routinely considered in defense calculations. . . . The likeliest and most dangerous future shocks will be unconventional. They will not emerge from thunderbolt advances in an opponent's military capabilities. Rather, they will manifest themselves in ways far outside established defense convention. Most will be nonmilitary in origin and character, and not, by definition, defense-specific events conducive to the conventional employment of the DoD enterprise. . . . They will rise from an analytical no man's land separating well-considered, stock and trade defense contingencies and pure defense speculation. Their origin is most likely to be in irregular, catastrophic, and hybrid threats of "purpose" (emerging from hostile design) or threats of "context" (emerging in the absence of hostile purpose or design). Of the two, the latter is both the least understood and the most dangerous.[47]

Narco-refugees, which would occur under each of the four scenarios, may be a strategic shock. Narco-refugees may become a "threat of context," which may also foreshadow potentially greater shocks to come for U.S. policymakers. Such shocks will mirror what other large refugee waves have created in other countries but will have features unique to the U.S.-Mexico relationship.

Like many refugee waves in other places, grievances from the country in con-flict can transfer to the host country. In the context of narco-refugees, the battle-fields of Mexican cartel violence may shift to the United States in ways previously not experienced. Once again, this would be due to geographic proximity. The heartland is adjacent to the U.S. states of California, Arizona, New Mexico, and Texas, and those states will likely experience the greatest influx of narco-refugees from neighboring heartland states. When placed together, the Mexican and U.S. states that share the border may form a zone of instability, a type of Waziristan that exists in northwest Pakistan that provides sanctuary for nonstate armed groups. Not all refugees are benign, and the longer they remain outside of their home coun-try and without adequate employment, there is the specter of narco-refugees using the United States as a safe haven for violent operations southbound. Beyond just perpetrating revenge killings, vigilante squads may form to return to Mexico in an attempt to "clear" towns of cartels and gangs. With easy access to guns in the United States, these squads could potentially conduct operations to establish con-ditions for the return of narco-refugees to Mexico. The questions are whether the U.S. government would seek to prevent or support such actions and what role the Department of Defense or DHS would play in such a scenario.

While the idea of U.S. border states serving as a safe haven for violent raids against cartels and gangs in Mexico may seem far-fetched at the moment, there are a number of elements that lend themselves to the plausibility of such a develop-ment. It is important to remember that LFM, the cartel that began the campaign of beheadings, is believed to have started as a vigilante group to combat drug deal-ers and kidnappers. Although not as sophisticated as LFM, the vigilante groups mentioned above, along with lynch mobs, have formed in Mexico and have acted against suspected kidnappers. In one instance, a mob blocked federal police from intervening to stop the beating of two suspected gang members.[48] The previously mentioned proliferation of armed groups in Mexico may spread to the United States. There would be little to stop vigilante communities from cropping up in the United States with the right mixture.

Part of the mixture already exists. The cases of Mexican mayors who reside in the United States demonstrate the ability to use the United States as a safe haven and to continue to make decisions from afar. "The advantage for them is that they cross the Rio Bravo (Rio Grande) and they are in their city hall or their home . . . or govern with the telephone in their hand."[49] The current use of temporary U.S. tourist and business visas by *inversionistas* has also been mimicked by reputed gang and cartel members.

Traditionally, when violence has spiked in Mexico, cartel figures have used U.S. cities such as Laredo, El Paso, and San Diego as rest and recreation spots, reasoning that the general umbrella of safety provided by U.S. law enforcement to those residing in the United States would protect them from assassination by their enemies. As bolder Mexican cartel hit men have begun to carry out assassinations on the U.S. side of the border in places such as Laredo, Rio Bravo, and even Dallas, the cartel figures have begun to seek sanctuary even deeper in the United States, thereby bringing the threat with them.[50]

Mexicans who seek to organize themselves in groups to forcibly return to Mexico can take advantage of this umbrella of protection. However, these groups would also be subject to attacks in the United States by cartels and gangs who seek to prevent them from interfering in their illicit operations. It is unlikely that U.S. citizens in these areas would idly watch these events; they may also form vigilante groups as counterweights.

Mexican groups arming themselves in the United States for attacks in Mexico would dramatically change the current understanding of spillover effects, as actions organized by those who fled high-intensity crime would add to the levels of violence back in Mexico. These levels would also increase the intensity of spillover, spill-back, and spill-around effects on U.S. interests. The result would be a sustainable dynamic of instability along the border that would be difficult for either the United States or Mexico to counteract effectively.

Stopping the Expansion of the Mosaic War

The future direction of Mexico's high-intensity crime as depicted in the previously described scenarios will force U.S. policymakers to consider approaches and options that have heretofore not been contemplated. However, the risk of an ever-expanding mosaic cartel war that more completely draws in the United States requires the thoughtful consideration of scenarios that may become reality. Any analysis and assessment of options to prevent or counter the worst features of the potential outcomes must be sober as well as bold. The uniqueness of a mosaic cartel war demands nothing less.

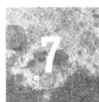

FINDING THE END
Recommendations and Responses

The potential outcomes for Mexico's mosaic cartel war as described in the previous chapter are grave and portend even graver loss and dislocation of life in Mexico than is currently occurring. The United States and Mexico will be inevitably bound together in whatever future scenario or scenarios unfold. Therefore, policy approaches will have to be carefully coordinated and implemented to avoid stoking more cartel violence, increasing the smuggling of drugs into the United States, and eroding Mexican governmental capacity. Uncoordinated and careless actions by either government run the risk of bringing to fruition the worst features of the scenarios discussed in the previous chapter or inadvertently bringing about some form of strategic shock. This risk makes the stakes for both countries exceptionally high and the execution of any set of policies very delicate.

When it comes to designing responses to prevent the occurrence of the scenarios' worst features, describing the clash among cartels, gangs, and the government in Mexico as a war of a different kind does not mean that a military option should follow. High-intensity crime with a hypercompetitive market at its core means that a military strategy is especially ill-suited to take on a mosaic cartel war. There is no military strategy that can defeat the law of supply and demand. This primary law of violent entrepreneurs' corporate logic is not conducive to being attacked based on military calculations of applying force to destroy the enemy. Declaring a war on violent entrepreneurs is one thing; defeating the source of their entrepreneurship with armed force is another. As this book has outlined, the mosaic cartel war in Mexico shares some common characteristics with all wars, such as organizational structures, leaders, fighters, battlefields, tactics, strategies, and counterstrategies. However, as demonstrated throughout the book, these characteristics take on different forms because of the criminal, rather than political, nature of the struggle. What is fundamentally a profound crisis of law and order in Mexico, with multiple social and political layers, brought about by economic conflicts over an illegal market cannot be solved with the application of military principles.

The vast, although partial, list of factors detailed in this book that make high-intensity crime complicated should give pause to anyone who believes that a military approach will bring it to a successful conclusion. The structural causes of the mosaic cartel war are many, including the signing of NAFTA; the loss of political power by the PRI; the confrontational approach to the cartels by the PAN; the number of cartels and gangs who exercise their corporate logic as violent entrepreneurs in a hyper-competitive illegal market; the allure of narco-cultura and machismo; the rise of women in cartels and gangs; the proximity to weapons markets; the insertion of former members of the military into cartel enforcement positions; the extent of geo-criminality; the institutional logic of government and law enforcement; the significance of being a hybrid node in regional drug trafficking networks; the fragility of Mexican democracy; and the continued use of the Mexican military for law enforcement. Each factor requires a response on its own merits, yet any single approach designed to tackle even one of these factors would be insufficient.

This book has rejected the thesis of the narco-insurgency/narco-terrorism school that sees the situation in Mexico as a form of low-intensity conflict. Not only is its analysis inconsistent with what is happening in Mexico, but it constructs cognitive frameworks for policymakers, distorting their options and forcing the discussion of responses into frameworks of counterinsurgency and counterterrorism. Andrew Bacevich's leeriness of using the term insurgency to describe the internal violence in Mexico is well-founded.

To frame the problem [in Mexico] as an insurgency almost necessarily invites a military response. I would be skeptical that a response that puts a primary emphasis on military power would be appropriate. The [U.S.] military that once claimed to have war figured out with "shock and awe" as a model now claims to have war figured out as counterinsurgency. Rather than treating different cases as distinctive, I think there is a tendency to apply the template, and today the template is counterinsurgency.[1]

This predisposition to view counterinsurgency as a strategic template to deal with high levels of internal violence has also manifested itself in the use of Colombia as analogy for the situation in Mexico. The use of the phrase "the Colombianization of Mexico" demonstrates how easy it is to succumb to such seduction.[2] Drug violence is a challenge to the state, no matter where or when it occurs, meaning that the institutions of government should be strengthened and bolstered. Not, however, in the same way that a counterinsurgency strategy would do so. Colombia's Democratic Security Policy (DSP) and the U.S. Plan Colombia are not the same as Mérida Initiative. The spine of the DSP is to bring areas that have long been beyond the authority of the government in Bogota due to the presence of various nonstate armed groups back under national administration. Often this has meant the use of military force against guerrillas. Rather than securing territory from insurgents, Mexico has a far more vexing problem—the territories that the government seeks to reclaim from cartel violence are cities that have been nominally under government control for many years. The Mexican government must vouch for those already in positions of power and authority who are ostensibly charged with combating narcotics trafficking and its associated violence in areas where drug cartels are most active. The use of the Mexican military notwithstanding, the country is still a federal system with a patchwork of competing legal authorities and jurisdictions that greatly complicates efforts to gain the upper hand against the cartels.

Ideally, any strategy would be long-term with the ultimate goal of closing Mexico's capacity gaps and function holes and reducing the U.S. demand for drugs. Counterinsurgency and counterterrorism are incongruent means to accomplish such goals. Adopting either as a strategic approach risks not just failure but the exacerbation of violence and the potential rupturing of positive relations between the United States and Mexico that are required for a host of other important issues unrelated to high-intensity crime, such as immigration, trade, and responses to pandemics. Operationally, counterinsurgency and counterterrorism approaches are also exceptionally thorny even in the proper context. For example, when it came to dealing with police responsibilities in Northern Ireland, an independent commission found that:

> We cannot emphasize too strongly that human rights are not an impediment to effective policing but are, on the contrary, vital to its achievement. Bad application and promiscuous use of its powers to limit a person's human rights—by such means as arrest, stop and search, house searches—can lead to bad police relations with entire neighborhoods, thereby rendering effective policing of those neighborhoods impossible.[3]

In the face of nearly daily atrocities occurring in Mexico and outgunned, feeble local police, the need for policymakers "to do something" is acute, making familiar templates of counterinsurgency and counterterrorism seductive choices.

Police may be put at risk and incapable of acting as core police in the event of not only insurgencies but of ordinary crime, in particular the organized trafficking of narcotics and people. . . . The great dilemma for policymakers, then, is how to meet shifting conditions of security without handicapping the opportunity for deploying core police who can win hearts and minds. In particular, should police themselves develop the capacity to undertake offensive operations against the perpetrators of violence or should these by left to the military?[4]

In Mexico, the government has not chosen to make local or federal police in violence-wracked areas into "little soldiers" or to have the armed forces implement a military strategy against the cartels. The United States has largely supported this delicate balance. However, the continued reliance on the military for nonmilitary purposes has led to a strategic stalemate for the government, which has been unable to breakup the cartels substantially enough to either reduce the rates of violence in portions of the country or to stem the amount of drug trafficking. In other cases where militaries have encountered a stalemate at the strategic level, the response has often been to ratchet up tactics in an effort to show progress. With the jump in the number of human rights abuse claims against the Mexican military, this may already be happening. It would be inconsistent to call oneself a democratic country if citizens are arbitrarily arrested or subjected to unreasonable force and if dissent is suppressed.[5] Ratcheting up tactical uses of the military in a situation of high-intensity crime carries with it the fatal risk that deep social divisions will emerge as the result of heavy-handed tactics, paving the way for a genuine insurgency to begin and increasing the danger of a fragmenting Mexican state.

Thus a conundrum appears to exist in this book—although it has used the term "war" to add analytical clarity, it may appear to be just as guilty as the narco-insurgency/narco-terrorism school by narrowing the policy options and predisposing policymakers toward selecting a military strategy with the active use of armed forces. However, a mosaic cartel war is a manifestation of high-intensity crime, which is a condition where violent entrepreneurs seek to prevail over one another and the state in a hypercompetitive illegal market in order to control it or a particular portion of it. High-intensity crime in the case of Mexico is a mosaic of several conflicts—cartels among each other, within cartels, cartels against the Mexican state, cartels and gangs against the Mexican people, and gangs versus gangs—occurring together in a number of locations for varied reasons related to drug trafficking. In fact, the narco-insurgency/narco-terrorism school focuses nearly exclusively on violent clashes between the cartels and the government; this is only one part of the mosaic and where the least amount of violence has occurred. Very scant attention is paid to the other portions of the mosaic. Therefore, to be more comprehensive and to avoid driving the discussion of options toward an approach that emphasizes military solutions, the concept of high-intensity crime is a better focal point on which to center policies for action.

Choosing to frame the issue around high-intensity crime does not lessen the significant security issues created by it. As discussed in the first chapter, high-intensity crime can lead to much greater levels of violence than low-intensity conflicts. Such violence is based on the corporate logic of the cartels that was detailed in chapter 2, and the importance of a particular territory—geo-criminality—was described in chapter 3. Additionally, chapter 4 covered the far-reaching and widespread effects of Mexico's drug-fueled violence on U.S. interests; chapter 5 discussed the complicated Mexican and U.S. responses to high-intensity crime, while chapter 6 outlined the dangerous outcomes if the violence continues or worsens. In many aspects, the concept of high-intensity crime makes tackling it a more nettlesome problem for decision makers.

Using a framework that addresses a complex form of criminality means that "strategies to tackle organized crime must take account of the social, economic, and political domains within which it operates."[6] By focusing on high-intensity crime, policies may be developed that avoid actions that will thicken the nexus where Mexico's institutional weaknesses intersect with the powerful U.S. demand for drugs. This is a tall order indeed, but a comprehensive strategy focused on key portions of high-intensity crime has a better chance of success than counterinsurgency and counterterrorism because it lowers the risks of misaligning a strategic goal with inappropriate approaches.

High-Intensity Crime and Legalizing Drugs

One suggested comprehensive approach that is not a military strategy is to legalize drugs. In essence, advocates of drug legalization believe that they are striking at the heart of what causes violence—legalization will bring order to a disordered market and remove the hypercompetitive nature of the market, thus nearly eliminating violent entrepreneurs as participants. Violence would diminish because the corporate logic of the cartels would become extinct.

When looking at Mexico and its high-intensity crime, legalization advocates generally agree that drug policy cannot be divorced from national security. They believe that the prohibition paradigm as manifested in the war on drugs is the main contributor to instability in Mexico. In contrast to the $18 billion and $39 billion spent annually on narcotics coming northward, the United States alone has spent more than $2.5 trillion over the past forty years in a war on drugs, yet drug use has remained constant, with ebbs and flows based on shifts in the types of drugs consumed. The only real change has been the rising levels of violence associated with the drug trade. In 2009, Director Gil Kerlikowske of the ONDCP (the "drug czar"), scrapped the phrase "the war on drugs" and sought to redirect efforts to demand reduction. This was not legalization or decriminalization, as a considerable proportion of federal counternarcotics budget was still aimed at supply side reduction, interdiction, and law enforcement. Prohibition is still the overarching framework under which drug demand is tackled in the United States. The argument of legalization advocates appears sound: prohibition does not work and is even counterproductive to U.S. national security interests. As long as strong demand continues under a paradigm of prohibition, there is a high likelihood that cartel violence in some degree will continue as well.

While seemingly logical, drug legalization as a way to bring Mexico's high-intensity crime to an end faces significant hurdles. First, the United States has played a leading role in the international prohibition of narcotics trafficking; it is highly unlikely that the United States would divest itself of its domestic policies then lead an international movement for legalization or strongly support the efforts of other nations to do so. Certain national governments of source countries may legalize the growth of certain drug crops, and other governments of demand countries may decriminalize the use of certain drugs, but the international prohibition of the trade itself will likely remain. It would take a massive, and nearly sudden, shift in attitudes to bring about the return of the legal commercialization of the narcotics trade. In fact, there is not a single country that has fully legalized the distribution and use of all narcotics. Legalization in the United States would do little to change the illegal status of the international trade of hard drugs produced from poppies, coca, and cannabis and synthetic chemicals.

The importance of Mexico's stance must also be added to the debate over legalization. If only one country retains prohibition against the drug trade while the neighboring country adopts more permissive laws, a type of narcotics-driven security dilemma will be created. Harsh restrictions do not lessen demand, and with increased risk, illicit trafficking into a more prohibitive environment to meet the market would be seductively lucrative. Meanwhile, in nations where drug consumption is legal, "drug tourists" from the country with harsh measures may swamp the more permissive state. Governments will be forced to either forego legalization efforts because they are being undermined or revert back to harsher enforcement measures in attempt to stem the tide of black market narcotics.

Second, it is unclear that legalization would lessen the pressures of a hypercompetitive market. A crucial policy question is whether legalization means commercialization along the lines of alcohol or cigarettes. Would private companies be permitted to produce, distribute, and market their narcotic products? Commercialization will lead to "lower prices, easier access, and heavy promotion."[7] The goal of commercial companies in a legal environment would be similar to that of violent entrepreneurs in an illegal environment—to get their product into as many, not as few, as hands possible. Even if certain drugs were legalized and commercialized, it is likely that governments in the name of public health and public safety would restrict the level of intoxicating and addictive chemicals present in a particular drug product. Controlling the level of intoxicant in a narcotic would likely lead back to the black market; people would look for drugs with higher concentrations of intoxicants. Thus, the dynamics for a hypercompetitive market would be set in motion once again.

Also, drug trafficking is a transnational business. Would existing trade agreements, such as NAFTA, be elastic enough to permit narcotics commerce or would new trade arrangements be required? In some ways, the global spread of cigarette smoking offers a preview of drug legalization and commerce. When the United States adopted more regulation of the cigarette industry, companies shifted their focus to overseas markets. Countries seeking to protect their own domestic cigarette industry and to limit cigarette smoking due to public health concerns were subjected to powerful lobbying in the WTO to allow overseas competition from American cigarette companies.[8] In addition, violent entrepreneurs have not been disengaged from the cigarette market because of the commercialization of nicotine. Cigarette smuggling and counterfeit cigarette manufacturing are activities carried out by organized crime and are subject to the pathologies of a hypercompetitive illegal market as well. The black market is alive and well for cigarettes, and smuggling across the Akwesasne Indian Reservation in Massena, New York, and Canada is one of the biggest and most violent problems for the U.S. Border Patrol on the northern border.

As far as reducing violence associated with a hypercompetitive market, legalization may not be effective. A Rand study on marijuana legalization found that in the short term, there could be additional violence resulting from at least three sources:

- Conflict between the current leaders and the dismissed personnel.
- Conflict within cartels. Even after the firing of excess personnel, the earnings of the leadership most likely will decline. One way a cartel

lieutenant might compensate for this is to eliminate his or her superior, generating internal violence from senior managers who become more suspicious in the face of the overall decline in earnings.

■ Conflict between cartels. The leadership of an individual cartel may try to maintain their earnings by eliminate rivals.[9]

The long-term prognosis of the study was more positive about reduction in violence associated with the marijuana trade in particular, but there were open questions about the strategic thinking of cartels and gang members "that appear to have a propensity for expressive and instrumental violence."[10] It is uncertain whether violence would return in the long-term in another hypercompetitive market.

This leads to a third problem with the legalization approach—as violent entrepreneurs, Mexican cartels may adapt their proficiency in violence to service any new dynamics that drug legalization brings. Cartels and gangs may choose to move into the market for prescription drugs. Prices for them are much lower in Mexico than in the United States, meaning that cartels could divert prescription drugs to compensate for the closure of any markets for narcotics caused by legalization. Or, as noted above, if there is not a coordinated trade agreement for legalized narcotics between the United States and Mexico, price margins may also create opportunities for the diverting of cheaper and more powerful drugs into the United States. The result may again be high-intensity crime because "in a world protected by the mafia, sellers compete, not by improving quality or by reducing prices but by acquiring more efficient violent skills in order to enlarge their share of the market."[11] Moreover, as seen in previous chapters, with well-established smuggling routes in place, cartels can turn their networks toward other illicit trade unrelated to drugs. Human trafficking, for example, is a lucrative trade whose profits are competitive with illicit narcotics. A captured money launderer belonging to LFM confessed to illegally exporting 1.1 million tons of iron ore last year to China, netting $42 million.[12] In another instance, the Mexican oil pipeline explosion that killed twenty-eight people in December 2010 was caused by drug gangs tapping the line to siphon petroleum for black market sales. Furthermore, there is evidence that Mexican cartels are diversifying into cyber crime such as fraud and identity theft. They still use violence by coercing and kidnapping computer programmers and engineers to help them perpetrate these schemes.[13]

Without overcoming these obstacles, the paradox of the drug trade and forms of organized violence will continue. Policymakers will continue to be forced to operate in this paradox and manage its more pernicious and dangerous effects. At best, the drug trade will decrease or continue at present levels and policy struggles will continue; at worst, the drug trade and its attendant violence will continue, with Mexico and the United States being challenged by increasingly powerful transnational criminal enterprises.[14]

Baseline Recommendations

If some form of drug legalization occurs, it is still many years and many tough decisions away. Although the war on drugs may have been dropped as a rhetorical phrase, this has not triggered new and differing patterns of behavior among drug traffickers and drug users. Clandestine smuggling, sale, and distribution by violent entrepreneurs are still the main characteristics of the contemporary drug trade. The policy dilemmas that this produces can only be managed, rather than solved in a conclusive or satisfactory manner. Managing an endemic social issue like crime sets it apart from traditional understandings of ending a war.

The following recommendations fully acknowledge the dilemmas but offer ways to form the contours of a more comprehensive approach to high-intensity crime in Mexico beyond legalization of the drug trade. These recommendations also include ways that the Mérida Initiative, or a successor policy, can be expanded to support the efforts that have already been undertaken by the United States and Mexico.

Avoid Further Militarization of the Situation in the Near Term

As mentioned previously, militaries with long-term and sustained exposure to counternarcotics operations invariably suffer from many forms of institutional corruption, from collusion with traffickers to abuses of power. However, there are other reasons not to increase the number of armed forces used along the border in particular. Given the proximity of violence to the U.S. border, long-term use of the Mexican army might lead to more border incursions and increases the potential for the accidental use of force. Deaths of U.S. law enforcement officers at the hands of Mexican soldiers or vice versa would have severe implications for both countries. The activation of the National Guard in border states contributes to these dangers. Having two militaries operating on either side of the border that may accidentally clash could diminish the necessary cooperation and good will needed for a mutually beneficial cross-border relationship. A violent exchange between the security forces on either side of the border may inject more hypercompetitive qualities into the market by creating a deeper reservoir from which traffickers draw recruits within Mexico and enticing more Americans to become straw purchasers and mules for the gun trade going south.

Cartels or gang members may even seek to provoke cross border violence between the two sides as a strategy to drive a wedge between the United States and Mexico or as an operational tactic to draw attention away from their plazas and toward the plazas of their rivals. By forcing the American administration to deploy more military assets to the border, cartels may be able to frustrate the American electorate and undermine the U.S. president's standing among those NGOs that support liberal immigration policy. These organizations will likely latch onto the deployment of the troops as targeting illegal immigrants more than targeting drug traffickers, placing additional political pressure on decision makers.

If Mexican decision makers feel the need to continue to use the armed forces to take on the cartels, they must be properly trained in law enforcement. This means an overhaul of the current training system, perhaps along the lines of the Italian model. The national police of Italy, along with military units that are tasked to tackle the Mafia, are trained in the same national academies. Gaining assistance from Italian counterparts would be useful for Mexico.

U.S. policymakers should also resist pressures to classify Mexican cartels as "foreign terrorist organizations" for a number of important reasons. First, doing so could put a strain on relations between the United States and Mexico because the Mexican government has not labeled the cartels as terrorist groups. If the United States labeled the cartels as terrorists without an agreement from Mexico, it would represent a step beyond where the Mexican government may be willing to go. Second, doing so may raise the profile and prestige of the cartels, giving them more prominence than they merit. Once again, this may create a rift with Mexico. Finally, the cartels are already vulnerable to a vast array of criminal punishments; "anti-terror measures would not have any practical effect against them in terms of U.S. law enforcement."[15] Simply put, classifying cartels as terrorist groups would add little to current countercartel efforts.

Strengthen the Mexican State and Civil Society

The weakness of the criminal justice system has created an environment of impunity for drug traffickers. When only 5 percent of crimes in Mexico are solved, the result is inevitably higher levels of crime and violence. Without punishment for criminality, the allure of cartel soft power that celebrates a criminal lifestyle becomes even more powerful, and thus community support for drug trafficking organizations is facilitated and strengthened. The danger is the emergence of grassroots populism in support of cartels, further thwarting Mexican state authority and policy approaches designed to constrain the violence. Building and reinforcing state institutions, particularly in the area of criminal justice, therefore, is critical to the destruction of the culture of impunity. Timing, however, is critical. In this connection, it is possible that a modus vivendi will be established among competing cartels along the lines of the pax narcotica scenario described in the previous chapter. This may occur particularly if they conclude that violence has become highly counterproductive and hurts profit levels. In the Russian experience of high-intensity crime, President Vladimir Putin's reassertion of state power in Russia succeeded because it came at a time when spheres of influence among the violent entrepreneurs had been clearly demarcated and a degree of stability and predictability had reemerged in Russia's criminal world. A similar window of opportunity might appear in Mexico in the next few years.

Strengthening the Mexican state and civil society is a long-term commitment, which means that the United States must view the Mérida Initiative as vital, enduring, and elastic. Policymakers in the United States should continue to fund the Mérida Initiative and focus on how to continue to institutionalize Calderón's reforms. With new leaders in Mexico, the Mérida Initiative must focus on institutions rather than personalities. It should also take into account the need to focus on reforming municipal institutions like police forces and do so with the same robustness as it does with Mexican federal institutions. Calderón's strategy of using the military as a substitute for federal police that, when trained in the right numbers, will take on core policing responsibilities in the most violence-prone states and localities is logical, and the United States was right to support it. However, local police forces constitute 90 percent of Mexico's law enforcement personnel and have been targeted most by plata o plomo schemes. Local police forces also have low educational standards. Most municipal police have elementary-level education. Of the fifty-eight police academies throughout Mexico, only twenty-five have started to implement educational standards for applicants.[16] The remaining academies do not have uniform standards on educational qualification. Overall, these academies produce officers who have limited exposure to institutional rule-of-law standards. These shortcomings in training stem, again, from a lack of funding for local police forces. Public safety insured at the local level is the most durable, therefore strategies and their implementation should be developed in states and localities with heavy support from the federal governments in Mexico City and Washington, D.C.

The recent failures of "safe corridors" in Juarez reflect the need to train and professionalize local police. After intensive patrols along two main boulevards, the military handed off these safe corridors to federal police who then turned over responsibility to municipal police in November 2010. Crime rose fivefold after the transition to the city, including the kidnapping of a Northern Arizona University professor.[17]

Be Aware of the Differences between Plan Colombia and the Mérida Initiative

The Mérida Initiative should not be seen as a type of Plan Colombia. As previously discussed, there are key differences in the cases of Mexico and Colombia. The long-running drug violence in Colombia has been perpetrated by differing actors in different international contexts. There was a unique international seam where Colombia fell that gave impetus to various U.S. responses; this cannot be replicated in the case of Mexico. During the Cold War, American support for counternarcotics operations was secondary to the anticommunist crusade. When the Clinton administration developed Plan Colombia in the aftermath of the Cold War, counterinsurgency operations were conducted under the cloak of counternarcotics operations. In the post-9/11 world, counternarcotics have been subsumed under counterterrorism. Each American president has been able to increase or decrease the relative profile of Colombia's struggle against drug traffickers based on the international environment of the time. The international environment was then used to justify funding from Congress. Mexico, in contrast, has not been a battlefield of international politics, meaning that American policymakers cannot adjust their strategies to earn support from Congress in the same ways as they did with Colombia. In fact, there is already some congressional balking at the cost of Mérida Initiative.[18] The long-term sustainability of such funding is an open question that cannot be answered by adjusting the role counternarcotics plays in other struggles that are tied to an international dimension. Ways to justify such spending will rest on how it will contribute to greater safety for U.S. citizens at home and the reliability of Mexico as a partner to achieve a reduction in violence and drug trafficking. This reliability is likely to be an abiding debate in the halls of Congress.

Mobilize Outrage against Drug Trafficking Violence

One of the difficulties in Mexico is that violence has increased without creating a sense of outrage. A lesson of Sicily's experience of high-intensity crime is that when the population is outraged and is mobilized against organized crime, the criminals become more vulnerable. The exceptionally violent killings of state prosecutors Giovanni Falcone and Paolo Borsellino by use of high explosives transformed public apathy and acceptance into overt animosity toward the Sicilian Mafia. This was subsequently translated into further measures by the government to dismantle well-established structures of collusion and corruption. Replicating this in Mexico is difficult: civil society is at an inherent disadvantage when trying to deal with uncivil society. Moreover in large parts of Mexico, trafficking is deeply embedded both economically and socially in ways that help to sustain support for the drug business. This is where the Mexican government has to work hardest to inject alternative economic stimulants that can sustain growth and wean people away from what in some areas is the only form of economic subsistence. "By boosting the economic returns for staying on the right side of the law, 'carrots' might then dramatically alter the cost-benefit calculation facing potential criminals."[19] The battle for wallets and pocketbooks in many respects supersedes battle for hearts and minds. It is also a battle, however, that needs to facilitate and empower cross-border ties between United States and Mexican border communities to combat narco-cultura and the narco-economy.

Concentrate Focus on Criminal Finances

The Mexican government is not going to gain an advantage against the cartels by merely adding more boots on the ground unless there are more accountants with spreadsheets combing over trails of money. As mentioned in chapter 1, the longevity of a group of violent entrepreneurs is more vulnerable to disruptions in their finances than insurgents or terrorists. "Targeting illicit funds is one of the most effective ways of dealing with drug trafficking."[20] Therefore, a higher priority also needs to be given to targeting the proceeds of drug trafficking. The cartels' money laundering capability remains virtually untouched largely because Mexico's weak civil-asset-seizure law requires a tie to a criminal case. Additionally, real estate, a favorite way to hide criminal proceeds, is registered at the state level in Mexico and faces weak scrutiny. In fact, until 2011 the only money laundering investigative organization was the Financial Intelligence Unit (FIU) within the office of the secretary of finance and public credit.[21] The Mexican attorney general's office created a special unit for financial analysis against organized crime in 2011 that is designed to reinforce the FIU and streamline investigations and prosecutions. The number of financial investigatory bodies should be increased and be expanded to the geo-criminal heartland states in particular. This should also include the placement of U.S. Treasury agents alongside their Mexican counterparts. Calderón's reforms to the financial system were stymied in the legislature but should be attempted again.

Mexico's economy is still largely based on cash transactions that are harder to track and monitor. However, this makes the interdiction of southbound bulk cash smuggling an important part of a strategy to attack cartel finances. U.S. law enforcement and intelligence assets should also be directed at those groups that specialize in the smuggling of hard currency to Mexico.

Think of Narco-Cities Rather than a Narco-State

Compared to Colombia, which was challenged by powerful insurgencies operating freely in large swaths of territory and by the successful co-option of political leaders, the challenge to the Mexican state is thornier. Much of the violence is confined to a few cities mostly in the geo-criminal heartland and a few in the geo-criminal rimland. Policymakers should include geographic factors into their policies and options. Policy options must focus not only on the most violent cities but also on those in which there is little violence. Containing the violence and preventing its spread to critical areas of the geopolitical core, especially the capital of Mexico City, is essential. Intelligence analysis should be aimed at understanding how patterns of drug trafficking and violence may shift. Policymakers should then develop proactive measures to contain these effects and, in doing so, focus on lower levels of state and local governments as described above.

Tackle Demand through Adjusting Priorities

Although legalization may not be the best approach to dealing with high-intensity crime, decriminalization of use may be a suitable policy adjustment. Rather than legalizing drugs, decriminalization means removing the criminal penalties for use and possession of a certain amount of narcotics. Portugal decriminalized usage and possession not above more than the average dose for ten days of use for an individual. One of the key reasons Portugal moved to decriminalization and harm reduction policies was the "resource drain imposed by the criminalization regime."[22] Funds used to pursue drug offenders were shifted to treatment facilities. The same may be considered in the United States. Additionally, funds that are used to prosecute and incarcerate drug users could be directed toward treatment and supplement law enforcement operations aimed at dealers and traffickers.

Work to Control Southbound Weapons Flow

U.S. constitutional guarantees of gun ownership mean that more comprehensive restrictions on gun purchases would be difficult to achieve. Deeper collaboration between the police forces of Mexico and the United States is a healthy step, but more needs to be done, and there is a substantial U.S. responsibility to act domestically. Renewing the assault weapons ban may help. However, current control measures are lackluster; "time-to-crime" ratio—the time from when a weapon is purchased in the United States until it is recovered at a crime scene in Mexico— has grown shorter. This indicates that a steady supply of weapons is easily making its way across the border despite attempts at tighter control. Focusing attention on gun shows and closing loopholes are also positive steps. "Federal firearms licensees should be required to report multiple sales of two or more firearms within thirty days, instead of the current five business day period. This recommendation would build on the ATF's recent proposal and allow it to track all bulk firearm purchases."[23] Such information on bulk purchases would help the ATF and local law enforcement identify and apprehend potential gun traffickers. Increasing public education campaigns at gun shows about the dangers and effects of straw purchasers can also be beneficial.

Empower Mexican Civil Society

There is no reason that each policy action should have a government face to it. Mexicans and Americans routinely and peacefully cross the border for cultural, social, and economic reasons; they are deeply affected by the violence and must not feel disempowered. Grants should be established to create programs that share stories about how a narco-cultura has negatively affected ordinary people. Speaking tours of schools on the U.S. side by those who have lost relatives to the violence as well as expanded public education programs about the role played by straw purchasers in the ongoing violence should be encouraged. Tourism offices and travel websites should also be encouraged to make their clients aware of the possibilities of being approached by drug smugglers and the penalties incurred if they participate.

Grants should also be directed toward empowering "citizen journalists." Mexicans in violence-prone areas have already been gravitating toward blogs and social network sites like Twitter to find news about drug violence and to plan their daily activities. Parents now often check Twitter to find out if there are any shootouts when and where they take their children to and from school. In order to compensate for the deficit in traditional journalism because of cartel attacks against members of the media, citizen journalists can provide valuable information on the acts of the cartels and gangs through blogs and social media. Professional journalists should also be afforded protection from cartel attacks. A robust and multifaceted media that keeps the spotlight on cartel actions can also strengthen a civic culture that stands against narco-cultura. This is also an area where the Mérida Initiative could be expanded to include funding for such measures.

Assess the Options for Dealing with Narco-Refugees

Policymakers need to consider options and choices to cope with an influx of Mexicans who leave their country out of fear for their safety. Making an immediate change in policy without an overall assessment of the situation in Mexico and taking into account the broader interests in a stable and positive U.S.-Mexico relationship is exceptionally delicate. To admit an increasing number of asylum seekers into the United States undermines the message that Mexico is safe for American businesses and that the Mexican government is strong enough to prevail against the cartels. Also, allowing Mexicans to claim asylum could potentially open a floodgate of migrants to the United States during a time when there is a very contentious national debate over U.S. immigration laws pertaining to illegal immigrants. On the other hand, to deny the claims of asylum seekers and return them to Mexico where they might very well be killed strikes at the heart of American values of justice and humanitarianism.

Policymakers may gradually come to determine what path asylum seekers would take as time unfolds. A change could be made based on conditions such as a steady but rising number of narco-refugees or intermittent surges in numbers. Policymakers may also want to consider a triggered response to such changes in Mexico that portend the previously discussed dire scenarios. Once again, those seeking asylum may be a signal of changes in the health of the Mexican state, like a rise in the numbers of certain types of key individuals: military members, federal politicians, and prominent business leaders.

A sudden mass exodus, however, would pose special problems. Any policy option and the timing of its implementation would be subjected to a number of questions that would need answers. Would the sheer volume of people in a short period of time require detention facilities where Mexicans would be held as the determination of their status unfolds; would they be allowed into the United States on special visas and under what restrictions (for example that they not travel farther than twenty-five miles north of the border and may not seek employment); would U.S. sponsors be allowed to host certain Mexicans? Finally, what conditions in Mexico would be favorable for narco-refugees to be repatriated when the violence subsides? Policymakers should be prepared to answer these questions, politically charged as they are, before any sudden wave of narco-refugees moves toward the U.S. border.

A Way Forward: High-Intensity Law Enforcement

With these baseline recommendations, a broader approach to crafting a strategy can be developed. While an immediate goal is the reduction of violence in Mexico and its associated effects, expediency should not be substituted for the creation of durable practices of legitimate institutions that serve law-abiding citizens in a democratic nation. To confront high-intensity crime, Mexico, with cooperation from the United States, should engage in "high-intensity law enforcement," which means providing multifaceted, multilayered, and focused public safety in a complex environment of law and order while doing so within strong constitutional boundaries. Rather than a military strategy that focuses on killing or capturing the enemy or a population-centric counterinsurgency campaign to secure the population from irregular fighters, the focus of high-intensity law enforcement is to bring criminal offenders to justice and prevent crime in the future.

This is not to suggest that the answer to Mexico's high-intensity crime is to merely flood the streets with more police officers and dispense with basic civil liberties that underpin a strong democracy. Strong, but not aggressive, policing is part of any response to high levels of crime. Mexico should not become a police state, or a state full of police, by virtue of churning out more law enforcement officers through its academies. In fact, the number of police officers is not a problem in Mexico. With 366 officers per 100,000 people, Mexico is better supplied than the United States, Britain, France, and Italy.[24] However, their distribution is uneven and provides significant gaps in law enforcement. With over 2,000 municipalities, Mexico's municipal police exist in only 335 municipalities. Of these 335 municipalities, 87 utilize 69 percent of the resources and manpower, leaving the remaining municipalities with only 30 percent of resources.[25] For example, as it stands now, there are not enough Mexican military or federal police to patrol the rugged terrain of Sonora and Chihuahua.[26] This effectively abdicates power to the Sinaloa cartel. Deterring crime rests on the ability of the police to "gather evidence, solve crime, and make arrests. Any measure of the cost of crime [on the part of a criminal] ultimately rests on this activity."[27] Reducing zones of impunity in the long run and sustaining their reduction can only be achieved through a noncorrupt police presence. Outgunned police may require the assistance of the military when attacked. But here, too, effective policing can play a role in tackling this issue by including better intelligence and investigative techniques aimed at preventing powerful weapons from falling into the hands of cartels and gangs.

High-intensity law enforcement is a comprehensive, long-term approach. It is an approach that addresses as many possible pieces of a mosaic problem with the goal of reducing drug-fueled violence to a manageable law and order problem, similar to organized crime in the vast majority of other countries. It is not a military strategy that sees victory and defeat as viable goals that end a war. Rather than accepting the current levels of violence as the new abnormal scenario that was out-lined in the previous chapter, high-intensity law enforcement seeks to return crim-inal violence to normal levels prior to its upswing after 2006. Such an approach includes development programs and economic investment in areas where cartels draw their recruits. If these programs are focused and tailored, they can aid in strengthening crime prevention in the long run. With persistence and creativity, this may lead to changes in civic culture that reject, or at least effectively resist, the allure of narco-cultura.

If combating Colombia's drug violence offers any lessons, it is the need for a long-term commitment to police and judicial approaches.

A close study of USG [U.S. government] involvement in Colombia reveals that a range of wide-scale and comprehensive efforts, which are the result of long years of trial and error, have been successful in developing Colombian LE [law enforcement] capabilities and RoL [rule of law] systems, and improv-ing governance. The Colombia example shows the value of a comprehensive, long-term commitment to a partner nation and highlights successes of years of involvement and increasingly well-integrated USG IA [interagency] efforts. Colombia also reveals the value of a HN [host nation] government taking the lead in developing its capabilities and running operations . . . and politi-cal will to make necessary changes within the HN domestic system.[28]

A long-term commitment to high-intensity law enforcement must be paired with Mexican willingness to the end the criminal-patronage networks in Mexico. There must be enough political will to break the links between traffickers and polit-ical figures. Without substantial weakening of the political-criminal nexus, any approach to tackle the cartels will be crippled from the outset, and the U.S. long-term commitment may be sapped.

Paradoxically, political will may be best generated if the cartels begin to target political leaders for violent reprisals. In essence, if cartel leaders break their links with politicians because individual cartel leaders see their political protectors as unable to get the government to stop pursuing them, then political leaders may begin to more forcefully target the cartels because they see no other option. As Luis Astorga explains, "If [violence] reaches members of the political and business elite, they can pressure the political class to act responsibly. . . . They would have to reveal those within their ranks—and they know who they are—who provide pro-tection in one way or another to certain groups in specific regions."[29] As seen with the rise of the PAN and Calderón's more confrontational stance, breaking the nexus more completely, may lead to another cycle of violence.

Political will, however, may be undermined through the infiltration of narco money in national elections. Bribes to state and local political figures involved in elections have been a mainstay of the Mexican political scene. National political figures have also been implicated in accepting tainted contributions and bribes. This may increase as cartels attempt to sway national elections in favor of candidates who are not as confrontational in their drug policies. The cartels may support candidates who are against extradition of Mexicans to the United States for drug crimes, for example. The human rights requirements under the Mérida Initiative may also open avenues for political platforms that emphasize nationalist and sovereignty issues that point to U.S. interference in Mexican affairs. Once again, cartels may encourage and support popular protests aimed at the military and the government.

A multinational layer must also be part of high-intensity law enforcement. Because drug violence has spill-around effects on U.S. interests and because drug trafficking has regional implications, countries from around the world can be involved in assisting the Mexican government. In fact, other countries such as the United Kingdom, France, Italy, Spain, and Colombia have had histories of implementing tough law enforcement reforms; such experiences and the expertise that they have generated in the intervening years can be of great benefit to Mexico in its current struggles. The third member of NAFTA, Canada, also has excellent resources that can be useful to Mexico; the Royal Canadian Mounted Police, for example, has a strong record of tackling money laundering that can also be used to assist Mexican authorities.

Strategic Options for High-Intensity Law Enforcement

Under a high-intensity law enforcement approach, a number of strategic options can be formulated and implemented. One strategy is multifaceted and tackles many cartels at once; another focuses on the geo-criminal territory of the cartels; another is sequential in its actions against the cartels. The options are a starting place for consideration; they are not mutually exclusive, and many elements of each option can be mixed and matched.

Mosaic Countercartel Strategy

A "mosaic countercartel strategy" would seek to weaken cartels simultaneously rather than sequentially. It was suggested in the preceding chapters that one of the lessons from Mexico's own experience of attacking the cartels over the years is the need to avoid creating instabilities and opportunities in the criminal world that encourage rather than discourage violence. In effect, it is necessary to adopt a broad countercartel strategy that incrementally weakens groups across the board but does not create major perturbations in the criminal world. Efforts should be made to create short rather than long vacancy chains and avoid asymmetric reductions in the power of one or two drug trafficking organizations. Long vacancy chains and asymmetric reductions make attractive targets for rivals to attack. The mosaic counter-cartel strategy will require substantial resources from the Mexican government, while the U.S. government will have to increase its support in order to compensate for any shortfalls in funding. Different strategies directed against different cartels should be done in parallel rather than done sequentially. The different strategies should be: elimination of Los Zetas, dismantling of BLO, delegitimizing LCT, shrinking Sinaloa, and containing Juarez, Gulf, and Tijuana.

The Mexican government should have a goal of eliminating Los Zetas. With their expertise in unconventional warfare, knowledge of the workings of the Mexican military, and skills in psychological operations, Los Zetas are the most likely group out of all the cartels to evolve into an insurgent or terrorist group. Therefore, its defeat is critical for the government in order to prevent such an occurrence. DDR projects aimed at Los Zetas would be of limited utility; integration of its members back into the Mexican armed forces may only corrupt them and undermine the rule of law in the long run. Surrenders of members of Los Zetas may be encouraged with the understanding that prosecutions would be followed by tailored sentences based upon information gained from members that leads to the further weakening of the group and its drug trafficking operations.

When it comes to the BLO, the strategy should be to dismantle the group. The BLO has been systematically disrupted over the years with arrests and deaths of key family members. This has led to divisions and more distant family members attempting to take the reins of the group. Continued pressure should be placed on the cartel in order to prevent its reconstitution. This may also lead to its absorption by another cartel. However, this may lead to a reduction in violence in areas that the BLO once controlled.

Because both LFM and LCT have a quasi-belief system that justifies many of their actions, it must be delegitimized. Although the number of killings decreased after the death of Nazario, many areas of Michoacán are still under the sway of LFM and LCT, and many Michoacanans do not believe the cartels will ever disappear. The director of a drug treatment center in the city of Apatzingan, Michoacán, stated that "nothing has changed. The narcos will never go away."[30] The supervisor of a local fire station said that he still must call an LCT representative to get permission to send ambulances to respond to calls.[31] The perception of LFM's and LCT's permanence must be challenged; the myth of their invincibility along with the power of their message must be seen by the community as illegitimate. The areas where LFM and LCT operate should be the focus of more community development programs and improved government services.

Much of the intercartel violence in the geo-criminal heartland was precipitated by the intrusions of the Sinaloa cartel. Government actions must be aimed at shrinking its presence in the heartland and reducing its influence in other parts of the country that overlap with more local cartels. Sinaloa leader Guzman's very ambitious attempt to extend his influence over other cartels and their territory must be rolled back. His aggressive forays into the geo-criminal heartland touched off much of the violence in Juarez and Tijuana. Shrinking the Sinaloa cartel's expansion may also have a similar effect in other places.

The remaining cartels of Juarez, Gulf, and Tijuana should be contained to the areas where they are currently located. Keeping violent entrepreneurs relegated to their traditional areas of operations has produced lowers levels of violence in other cases of high-intensity crime. The yakuza wars in 1950s Japan ended when each side in the conflict returned to their traditional spheres of influence. Containing the Juarez, Gulf, and Tijuana cartels to their spheres of influence may induce calm and create enough stability for the return of well-trained and vetted police. Over time, this may lead to tackling the cartels more aggressively at a later stage.

Heartland Strategy

Because the greater proportion of cartel and gang violence occurs in the heartland and because the United States is more focused on acts of violence along the border, policymakers may choose a strategy that centers on the geo-criminal heartland. Rather than tackling all the cartels at once as described in the mosaic countercartel strategy, a heartland strategy would take on the cartels who are based in the six northern Mexican states of Baja California, Sonora, Chihuahua, Coahuila, Nuevo Leon, and Tamaulipas. This strategy would be more than simply containing the cartels that are indigenous to the area. It would be a comprehensive program that seeks to close the gap between the geo-criminal heartland and the geopolitical core by making the states and cities in the geo-criminal heartland higher priorities for federal funding.

Focusing law enforcement efforts more strongly on the cartels and gangs in the region should only make up part of the strategy; policymakers should also create

a development program that focuses on the region as a whole. "For all the lia-
bilities of security- and interdiction-focused efforts, they remain vital compo-
nents of any comprehensive counterdrug program. Economic development and
political reform cannot exist in a context of violent anarchy, any more than internal order can be sustained if these deeper problems remain unresolved."[32] The
ability to address economic inequality and social alienation in the geo-criminal
heartland will go a long way in removing many of the drivers of drug trafficking
and its attendant violence. The "miracle of Medellin" in one of Colombia's most
violent cities demonstrates the possibility of reducing drug homicides by focusing on security and development in a violence-wracked area. In the 1980s and
1990s, Medellin had a murder rate nearly twice as high as present-day Ciudad
Juarez; now it has only one-fifth of what it was at its height in the 1990s.[33] For
Mexico, more will be needed; micro-loan programs, vocational training, drug
abuse treatment, and reintegration of reformed gang members should all be
included in this strategy.

Such a strategy may become subject to the balloon effect where cartels and gangs
merely shift their operations to areas that are less resistant to their presence and
activities. Preventive efforts should be started in coastal areas of the rimland in particular, which can be used to transport drugs by sea.

Zeta First Strategy

As described in the mosaic countercartel strategy, Los Zetas are the greatest armed
threat to the Mexican government because of their expertise and proficiency in
military tactics and operations. They were the first group of enforcers to bring their
military expertise to intercartel conflicts and they are also a group that has most
aggressively and directly confronted the Mexican military in pitched battles. But
they have lost the majority of these confrontations. Their weakness in the face of
armed battles makes their operational arm more vulnerable to traditional military
tactics. One finding by H. R. Friman in his study of drug markets and violence was
"that the more successful state enforcement efforts are in disrupting the trafficking
organization, the shorter the period of violence between the targeted organization
and the state, but at the risk of increased violence between contending groups seeking to fill the gap."[34] With Los Zetas's inability to wrest a large portion of the drug
trade from the Gulf cartel and others, focusing on dismantling Los Zetas first may
not create large vacuums that leads rivals to fight to fill. In fact, the cartels in the
New Federation may extend their cooperation in the absence of Los Zetas to divvy
up the spoils.

Rival cartels, like those in the New Federation, may even choose to assist the government with intelligence on Los Zetas's operations. This may play into the accidental narco scenario. However, the government, upon sufficiently weakening or dismantling Los Zetas, may then turn its attention to taking on the other cartels, perhaps using the other two strategies as described in this chapter. In some ways, this strategy mirrors the Colombian government's strategy to more strongly go after the Medellin cartel because of Pablo Escobar's escalating violence and then focus on the Cali cartel after the death of Escobar and the destruction of his organization.

Those involved in implementing a strategy must guard against colluding with rival cartels. The temptation to gain more intelligence from criminal sources can have a corrupting effect on police and investigators. Pervasive collusion would lead to an accidental narco scenario and significantly undermine the legitimacy of the Mexican government's actions. Significant attention must be paid to mitigating this risk.

Conclusion: High-Intensity Law Enforcement and the Future of Mexico

High-intensity law enforcement has the familiar contours of the Mérida Initiative, but it is both more expansive in the resources that are required and more focused on specific functional and geographic areas where it can be implemented. High-intensity law enforcement is an imperfect approach to high-intensity crime and the mosaic cartel war that it has fueled. The approach will undoubtedly lead to many frustrations as it is implemented. "Even the flattest, most fluid enforcement networks still operate within the bounds of law and bureaucratic responsibility; trafficking networks do not. For this reason, enforcement networks will remain taller, more centralized, and less agile than their illicit adversaries."[35] Because it is implemented by a government in cooperation with another government, both of which are democracies, flexibility and swiftness will not be chief characteristics of high-intensity law enforcement. Nonetheless, high-intensity law enforcement offers the best chance of forestalling the emergence of the dangerous scenarios—new abnormal, accidental narco, pax narcotica, or Zeta state—that may create a strategic shock for the United States.

The struggle against Mexico's violent entrepreneurs will be long and uncertain. As entrepreneurs of illegal business, Mexican cartels will continue to innovate in an effort to survive and rake in illicit profits. If such criminal innovation is to be blunted, the mutually reinforcing dynamic that has fueled much of the violence in Mexico must be replaced with mutually reinforcing cooperation that is supported by trust on both sides. Although flexibility and swiftness may not be hallmarks of high-intensity law enforcement, fair and durable institutions that dispense justice will be. Hopefully, the chief result will be a more peaceful Mexico and a thriving, beneficial relationship with the United States.

NOTES

Chapter 1. The Outbreak: The Wars Begin

1 James McKinley, "Two Sides of a Border: One Violent, One Peaceful," *New York Times*, January 22, 2009, http://www.nytimes.com/2009/01/23/us/23elpaso.html.

2 Nick Miroff, "Mexico Hopes $270 Million in Social Spending Will Help End Juarez Drug Violence," *Washington Post*, August 12, 2010, http://www.washingtonpost.com /wp-dyn/content/article/2010/08/11/AR2010081106253.html.

3 The term "cartel" is also the subject of much debate. Many U.S. governmental agencies and scholars prefer the term "drug trafficking organization" (DTO) over cartel. DTO as a term more strongly links the product that a group sells for profit while a cartel is able to control production and prices through collusion with other producers and suppliers. Rather than resolve this debate, for the purposes of this book, cartel and DTO will be used as equivalent terms.

4 John Burnett, "Sheriff to Texas Border Town: 'Arm Yourselves,'" National Public Radio, April 9, 2010.

5 Fred Burton and Scott Stewart, "Mexican Cartels and the Fallout from Phoenix," Stratfor, July 2, 2008, www.stratfor.com/weekly/mexican_cartels_and_fallout _phoenix.

6 U.S. Immigration and Customs Enforcement, "Statement of Marcy Forman, Director," March 1, 2006, www.ice.gov/doclib/pi/news/testimony /060301homelandpdf.

7 Doris Gomora, "Se dispara peticion de asilo de mexicanos en EU," *El Universal*, November 7, 2011, http://www.eluniversal.com.mx/notas/806794.html.

8 Philip Sherwell, "Mexican Drug Wars Force Police to Claim Asylum in U.S.," *London Daily Telegraph*, April 11, 2009, www.telegraph.co.uk; Alfonso Chardy, "Mexicans Caught in Drug War Get U.S. Asylum,"www.azcentral.com, April 5, 2010, http://www.azcentral.com/news/articles/2010/04/05/20100405mexico -asylum0405.html.

9 Barry McCaffrey, "After Action Report—Visit Mexico—5–7 December 2008," 4.

10 Interview with President Obama by regional reporters, March 12, 2009, http://www.enewspf.com/index.php?option=com_content&view=article&id=6317 :interview-of-president-obama-by-regional-reporters&catid=1&Itemid=88889791.

11 Andrew Selee, David Shirk, and Eric Olson, "Five Myths about Mexico's Drug War," *Washington Post*, March 28, 2010.

12 Mark Potter, "Drug War 'Alarming' U.S. Officials," msnbc.com, June 25, 2008, http://worldblog.msnbc.msn.com/archive/2008/06/25/1166487.aspx.

13 Sarah Miller Llana, "Mexican Workers Send Less Cash Home from U.S.," *Christian Science Monitor*, January 28, 2009, http://www.csmonitor.com/World/Americas /2009/0128/p25s20-woam.html.

14 Secretario de Turismo, Mexico, "Mexico's International Tourism Revenues Reach Historic High," press release, March 7, 2007, http://www.1888pressrelease.com /mexico-s-international-tourism-revenues-reach-historic-high-pr-8r82w4eo15.html.

15 "Mexican Crimewave: America's Southern Neighbor Is Succumbing to Bloody Anarchy," timesonline.co.uk, September 1, 2008, http://www.timesonline.co.uk /tol/comment/leading_article/article4647962.ece.

16 Selee, Shirk, and Olson, "Five Myths."

17 CNN, "American Morning," (transcript), aired July 29, 2009, http://transcripts.cnn.com/TRANSCRIPTS/0907/09/ltm.01.html.

18 Ryan Grim, *This Is Your Country on Drugs* (Hoboken, NJ: Wiley and Sons, 2009), 104.

19 Ibid.

20 Julian Borger and Jo Tuckman, "Blood Brothers," *London Guardian*, March 15, 2002, http://www.guardian.co.uk/world/2002/mar/15/mexico.julianborger. Thanks to Ms. Helen Lardner for the source.

21 Luis Astorga, "Drug Trafficking in Mexico: A First General Assessment," UNESCO Discussion Paper No. 36, http://www.unesco.org/most/astorga.htm.

22 Hal Brands, *Mexico's Narco-Insurgency and U.S. Counterdrug Policy* (Carlisle Barracks, PA: Strategic Studies Institute, 2009), 6.

23 Shannon O'Neill, "The Real War in Mexico," *Foreign Affairs*, July/August 2009, 65.

24 Roy Godson, "Political-Criminal Nexus: Overview," in *Menace to Society*, ed. Roy Godson (New Brunswick, NJ: Transaction Publishers, 2003), 5.

25 Voice of America News, "Mexico Promete Luchar La 'Madre de Todas Las Batallas' Contra El Narcotrafico,"January 22, 2005, www.voanews.com/spanish/archive /a-2005-01-22-2-1.cfm?renderforprint=1&&TEXTMODE=1&CFID=70719036 &CFTOKEN=37020507.

26 David Luhnow and Jose de Cordoba, "The Perilous State of Mexico," *Wall Street Journal Online*, February 21, 2009, http://online.wsj.com/article/SB123518102536038463.html.

27 Ruben Aguilar and Jorge Castaneda, *El Narco: La Guerra Fallida* (Mexico, DF: Punto de Lectura, 2009), 13. Translated from "la razon primordial de la declaracion de la guerra del 11 diciembre de 2011 fue politica: lograr la legitimacion supuestamente perdida en lasurnas."

28 O'Neill, "The Real War in Mexico," 77.

29 Marcelo Bergman, "Creating New Soldiers in Mexico's Drug War," foreignpolicy.com, May 17, 2010, www.foreignpolicy.com/articles/2010/05/17 /creating_new_soldiers_in_mexico_s_drug_war.html.

30 Ibid.

31 Mitchel Roth and Murat Sever, "The Kurdish Workers Party (PKK) as Criminal Syndicate,"*Studies in Conflict and Terrorism* (2007), 903.

32 Brands, *Mexico's Narco-Insurgency*, 4–5.

33 Adam Entous and Nathan Hodge, "U.S. Sees Heightened Threat in Mexico," *Wall Street Journal*, September 10, 2010.

34 Sylvia Longmire and John Longmire IV, "Redefining Terrorism: Why Mexican Drug Trafficking Is More than Just Organized Crime," *Journal of Strategic Studies* (November 2008), 37.

35 Lincoln B. Krause, "The Guerrillas Next Door," *Low Intensity Conflict and Law Enforcement* (Spring 1999).

36 Guy Lawson, "The War Next Door," Rollingstone.com, November 13, 2008, http://www.militaryphotos.net/forums/showthread.php?145209-The-War-Next-Door.

37 Robert J. Bunker, "Strategic Threat: Narcos and Narcotics Overview," *Small Wars and Insurgencies* (March 2010), 10.

38 Max Manwaring, A *"New" Dynamic in the Western Hemisphere Security Environment* (Carlisle Barracks, PA: Strategic Studies Institute, 2009), 2.

39 John Burnett and Marisa Peñaloza, "Mexico's Drug War: A Rigged Fight," National Public Radio, May 19, 2010, http://www.npr.org/templates/story/story.php?storyId =126890838.

40 Diego Gambetta, *The Sicilian Mafia* (Cambridge, MA: Harvard University Press, 1993), 7.

41 Malcolm Beith, "Are Mexico's Drug Cartels Terrorist Groups?" slate.com, April 15, 2010, http://www.slate.com/toolbar.aspx?action=print&id=2250990.

42 Michael Kenney, *From Pablo to Osama* (University Park: Pennsylvania State University Press, 2007), 9.

43 Audrey Kurth Cronin, "How Al Qaeda Ends," *International Security* (Summer 2006), 9.

44 Pino Arlacchi, "The Dynamics of Illegal Markets," in *Combating Transnational Crime*, ed. Phil Williams and Dimitri Vlassis (Portland, OR: Frank Cass, 2001), 9.

45 Thanks to Col. Eric Duke of the U.S. Army for this description.

46 Loretta Napoleoni, *Modern Jihad: Tracing the Dollars behind the Terror Networks* (Sterling, VA: Pluto Press, 2003), 165.

47 John Mueller, *Remnants of War* (Ithaca, NY: Cornell University Press, 2004), 6. See also Graham Turbiville, "Preface" in *Global Dimensions of High Intensity Crime and Low Intensity Conflict*, ed. Graham Turbiville (Chicago: University of Illinois, 1995), 7. Turbiville describes high-intensity crime as a condition that emerged in some

countries after the Cold War where "security problems that had in the past been driven by ideological, political, or other imperatives, now have strong criminal motivations *as well.* . . . To a growing extent, organized crime is providing an alternative means of support, as well as a seductive source of personal, criminal profit that *transforms ideological or political fervor.*" (Emphasis added.)

48 This is a twist on the adage from Mitchel Roth and Murat Sever, "The Kurdish Workers Party (PKK) as Criminal Syndicate," *Studies in Conflict and Terrorism* (2007), 902.

49 H. Richard Friman, "Drug Markets and the Selective Use of Violence," *Crime, Law, and Social Change* (September 2009), 287.

50 Brands, *Mexico's Narco-Insurgency,* 11.

51 Ed Vulliamy, "Killing for Kudos," *London Guardian Online,* February 7, 2010, http://www.guardian.co.uk/world/2010/feb/07/mexico-drug-war.

52 Mueller, *Remnants of War,* 86.

53 R. T. Naylor, "Violence and Illegal Economic Activity," *Crime, Law, and Social Change* (September 2009), 232.

54 Tom Farer, "Conclusion: Fighting Transnational Organized Crime," in *Transnational Organized Crime in the Americas,* ed. Tom Farer (New York: Routledge, 1999), 289.

55 Jorg Raab and H. Brinton Milward, "Dark Networks as Problems," *Journal of Public Administration Research and Theory* (October 2003).

56 Vadim Volkov, *Violent Entrepreneurs* (Ithaca, NY: Cornell University Press, 2002), 27–28.

57 Gambetta, *The Sicilian Mafia,* 2.

58 Peter Drucker, *Innovation and Entrepreneurship* (New York: Harper and Row, 1985), 29–36.

59 Ibid., 226.

60 Peter Reuter, "Systemic Violence in Drug Markets," *Crime, Law, and Social Change* (September 2009), 275.

61 Phil Williams, "The International Drug Trade," in Turbiville, *Global Dimensions of High Intensity Crime and Low Intensity Conflict,* 162.

62 R. T. Naylor, 236. "Selling crack cocaine is more likely to be associated with violence than peddling counterfeit Louis Vuitton handbags,"(235).

63 Bergman, "Creating New Soldiers in Mexico's Drug War."

64 "The Long Game," *Newsweek,* March 24, 2010, http://www.newsweek.com/2010/03/23/the-long-game.html.

65 Bergman, "Creating New Soldiers in Mexico's Drug War."

66 Federico Varese, *The Russian Mafia* (Oxford, UK: Oxford University, 2001), 190.

67 Borger and Tuckman, "Blood Brothers."

68 Nacha Cattan, "Fed Up with Plague of Kidnappings, Mexicans Turn to Mob Justice," *Christian Science Monitor,* September 22, 2010, http://www.csmonitor.com /World/Americas/2010/0922/Fed-up-with-plague-of-kidnappings-Mexicans-turn -to-mob-justice.

69 Richard Marosi, "A Tijuana Blood Bath," *Los Angeles Times*, October 6, 2008, http://articles.latimes.com/2008/oct/06/world/fg-arellano6.

70 Kenney, *From Pablo to Osama*, 10.

71 David Luhnow and Jose de Cordoba, "War on the Other Terror," *The Australian*, February 23, 2009, 7.

72 *The National Security Strategy of the United States of America* (Washington, DC: Government Printing Office, 2010), 42.

73 Grim, *This Is Your Country on Drugs*, 16.

74 Antonio Castelan, "Drug Cartel Members Kidnapping People in San Diego County," www.sandiego6.com, October 9, 2009, http://www.sandiego6.com/news/local/story/Drug-Cartel-Members-Kidnapping-People-in-San/VBWJH-_0I0y5U6o4zt8VTg.cspx.

Chapter 2. The "Warriors": Cartels and How They Fight

1 Robert Schoenberg, *Mr. Capone* (New York: Harper Collins, 1992) as quoted in Raymond Fisman and Miguel Edward, *Economic Gangsters* (Princeton, NJ: Princeton University Press, 2008), 5.

2 Pamela Bunker, Lisa Campbell, and Robert Bunker, "Torture, Beheadings, and Narcocultos," *Small Wars and Insurgencies* (March 2010), 150.

3 KBPS, "Border Battle: Bringing Home the Drug War, Glossary," accessed July 3, 2010, http://www.kpbs.org/news/border-battle/, quoted in Bunker, Campbell, and Bunker, "Torture, Beheadings, and Narcocultos."

4 R. T. Naylor, "Violence and Illegal Economic Activity," 241.

5 United States Department of Health and Human Services, results from the 2009 National Survey on Drug Use and Health, September 2010, http://www.oas.samhsa.gov/NSDUH/2k9NSDUH/2k9ResultsP.pdf.

6 Robert Bunker, "Strategic Threat: Narcs and Narcotics Overview," 17.

7 Ibid.

8 Ibid., 18.

9 Interview with Matt Stofolano (Chief Park Ranger of Coronado Memorial National Park, Arizona), December 9, 2010.

10 Jana Schroeder, "Mexico's Youngest Assassins," *Homeland Security Today* (March 2011), 28.

11 David Luhnow and Jose de Cordoba, "The Perilous State of Mexico."

12 Bunker, Campbell, and Bunker, "Torture, Beheadings, and Narcocultos," 150.

13 Phil Williams, "Illicit Markets, Weak States, and Violence: Iraq and Mexico," *Crime, Law, and Social Change* (September 2009), 325.

14 Friman, "Drug Markets and the Selective Use of Violence," 286.

15 Tony Payan, *The Three U.S.-Mexico Border Wars* (Westport, CT: Praeger Security International, 2006), 43–44.

16   Peter Reuter, remarks at the Migration Policy Institute, Washington, DC, February 18, 2009.

17   Diego Gambetta, *Codes of the Underworld* (Princeton, NJ: Princeton University Press, 2009), 30.

18   For example, a body that was dumped in Michoacán included a note that stated, "To those who don't believe it and don't have loyalty, greetings." William Finnegan, "Silver or Lead?" *The New Yorker*, May 31, 2010, 43.

19   Peter Reuter, "Systemic Violence in Drug Markets," 276.

20   Richard Friman, "Forging the Vacancy Chain," *Crime, Law, and Social Change* (December 2004).

21   "El Pacto del cartel del Golfo y Beltran," *El Universal*, May 19, 2008, http://www.eluniversal.com.mx/nacion/159611.html.

22   Gambetta, *Codes of the Underworld*, ix.

23   "Drug Cartel in Mexico Killing Street Dealers," azcentral.com, June 18, 2009, http://www.azcentral.com/news/articles/2009/06/18/20090618DrugWarMexico.html; "Cartel Stitches Victim's Face on Soccer Ball," msnbc.com, January 8, 2010, http://www.msnbc.msn.com/id/34774234/ns/world_news-americas/.

24   William Booth, "Mexican Cartels Send Messages of Death," msnbc.com, December 4, 2008, www.msnbc.com/id/2804515/print/1/displaymode/1098.

25   Ibid. (Emphasis added.)

26   Thomas Schelling, *Arms and Influence* (Westport, CT: Greenwood Press, 1977).

27   Associated Press, "Cartels Pay Corrupt Cops $100 Million a Month," *Borderland Beat*, August 9, 2010.

28   Maria de la Luz Gonzales, "Suman 10 mil 475 ejecuciones en esta administracion: PGR," *El Universal*, March 25, 2009, http://www.eluniversal.com.mx/nacion/166613.html.

29   Luhnow and Cordoba, "War on the Other Terror."

30   Letizia Paoli, "Criminal Fraternities or Criminal Enterprises?" in *Combating Transnational Crime,* ed. Phil Williams and Dimitri Vlassis (Portland, OR: Frank Cass, 2001), 100.

31   See Gambetta, *Codes of the Underworld*, 11–15.

32   Vuillamy, "Killing for Kudos."

33   Viridiana Rios, "Mexican Assassins on the Cheap," International Relations and Security Network, October 11, 2010, http://www.isn.ethz.ch/isn/Current-Affairs/ISN-Insights/Detail?lng=en&id=122286&contextid734=122286&contextid735=122282&tabid=122282.

34   "Chavez-Chavez Denies Acts of Terrorism, Sedena Still Deciding,"*El Diario Online*, July 17, 2010, www.diario.com.mx.

35   Carolyn Nordstrom, *Global Outlaws* (Los Angeles: University of California Press, 2007), 152.

36   Sam Quinones, "State of War,"*Foreign Policy* (March/April 2009), 78.

37 Elijah Wald, *Narcocorrido* (New York: Rayo, 2002).

38 See for example, "Mexican Singer Killed after Denying His Murder," BBC News, June 28, 2010, http://news.bbc.co.uk/2/hi/world/latin_america/10429934.stm; "Abducted Mexican Singer Strangled," BBC News, December 4, 2007, http://news.bbc.co.uk/2/hi/americas/7126594.stm; and Hector Tobar, "Mexican Pop Star, Manager Gunned Down," *Los Angeles Times*, November 26, 2006, http://articles.latimes.com/2006/nov/26/world/fg-mexdrugs26.

39 Matt Davis, "Jesus Malverde Legend Continues," *Portland Mercury*, May 28, 2009, http://blogtown.portlandmercury.com/BlogtownPDX/archives/2009/05/28/jesus -malverde-legend-continues.

40 D.E. Campbell, "A Saint for Lost Souls," *Foreign Policy* (May/June 2010), 34.

41 Jason Beaubien, "Saint or Sinner?" National Public Radio, April 13, 2009, http://www.npr.org/templates/story/story.php?storyId=102928118.

42 Vulliamy, "Killing for Kudos."

43 Ibid.

44 Instituto Nacional De Estadistica y Geografia, "Población total por grupos quinquenales de edad segúnsexo, 1950 a 2005," accessed on July 5, 2010, http://www.inegi.org.mx/inegi/default.aspx.

45 International Labour Office, "Mexico: Rising Unemployment, Higher Informal Sector Employment and Reduced Hours of Work," G20 Statistical Update, G20 Labor and Employment Minister Meeting, Washington, DC, 2010.

46 Reuter, remarks at the Migration Policy Institute.

47 George Grayson, *Mexico: Narco-Violence and a Failed State?* (New Brunswick, NJ: Transaction Publishers, 2009), 294.

48 Special thanks to Colonel Lorna Mahlock USMC for her contribution to this section.

49 Sedena Statistics, http://www.websitetrafficspy.com/www.sedena.gob.mx.

50 Associated Press, "Mexico Drug Violence Has Killed over 28,000 since 2006,"August 3, 2010.

51 Dianne Feinstein, Charles Schumer, and Sheldon Whitehouse, *Halting U.S. Firearms Trafficking to Mexico* (report to the U.S. Senate Caucus on International Narcotics Control, June 2011), 6.

52 Ibid.

53 James McKinley Jr., "U.S. Gun Dealers Arming Mexican Drug Cartels," *New York Times*, December 6, 2009, http://www.nytimes.com/2009/02/26/world/americas /26iht-border.4.20459692.html.

54 Scott Stewart, "Mexico: The Struggle for Balance," Stratfor, April 8, 2010, http://www.stratfor.com/weekly/20100407_mexico_struggle_balance.

55 Vuillamy, "Killing for Kudos."

56 Tony Payan as quoted in Booth, "Mexican Cartels Send Messages of Death."

57 The names of the founders of the seven cartels are compiled from borderlandbeat.com and borderviolenceanalysis.typepad.com while being verified against the information

provided by the National Drug Intelligence Center, Office of National Drug
Control Policy, Department of State, Department of Justice, and Stratfor.

58 "Tracking Mexico's Drug Cartels," Stratfor, December 11, 2008, www.stratfor.com
/theme/tracking_mexicos_drug_cartels.

59 Scott Stewart and Alex Posey, "Mexico: The War with the Cartels in 2009," Stratfor,
December 9, 2009, http://www.stratfor.com/weekly/20091209_mexico_war_cartels
_2009.

60 George Grayson, *Mexico: Narco-Violence and a Failed State?*, 84.

61 Ibid.

62 "Vicious Killings Escalate in Mexico Drug War," Reuters, October 7, 2008,
http://www.reuters.com/article/idUSN07366271.

63 Sandra Dribble, "Tijuana Violence Slows, Drops from Spotlight," *San Diego Union
Tribune*, April 26, 2010, http://www.signonsandiego.com/news/2010/apr/26/tijuana
-violence-slows-drops-out-of-spotlight/.

64 Jeremy Roebuck, "Authorities: Gulf Cartel, Zetas Gang Up on Each Other as Their
Arrangement Dies," *Rio Grande Monitor*, March 10, 2010, http://www.themonitor.com
/articles/gulf-36258-arrangement-reynosa.html.

65 Ibid.

66 "Mexico, the New Kingpins Rise," Stratfor, February 22, 2005.

67 Grayson, *Mexico,* 72.

68 Booth, "Mexican Cartels Send Messages of Death."

69 Alfredo Carchado, "Drug War Clashes between Gulf Cartel and Zetas May Escalate,"
Dallas Morning News, March 1, 2010, http://www.dallasnews.com/sharedcontent
/dws/dn/latestnews/stories/030110dnintdrugwar.416aff8.html.

70 "Gulf Cartel Goes Public on Break-Up with Former Allies," Deutsche Presse Agentur,
March 9, 2010, http://www.monstersandcritics.com/news/americas/news/article
_1539731.php/Gulf-Cartel-goes-public-on-break-up-with-former-allies-Los-Zetas.

71 "Formal Prision al asesino de 'El Pollo,'" *Notimex*, January 4, 2004,
http://www.esmas.com/noticierostelevisa/mexico/416169.html.

72 John Burnett, Marisa Peñaloza, and Robert Benincasa, "Mexico Seems to Favor
Sinaloa Cartel in Drug War," National Public Radio, July 24, 2010,
http://www.npr.org/templates/story/story.php?storyId=126906809.

73 Bruce Livesey, "Drug Cartels and the Mexican Military," *Vancouver Sun*, July 17,
2010, http://www.vancouversun.com/news/Drug+cartels+Mexican+army/3290794
/story.html.

74 "Mexican Police Free Reporters Nabbed by Drug Gang," msnbc.com, August 1,
2010, http://www.msnbc.msn.com/id/38504467/ns/business-media_biz/.

75 Sylvia Longmire, "TCO 101: The Cartel del Pacifico Sur," *Mexico's Drug War* (blog),
accessed on July 27, 2010, http://borderviolenceanalysis.typepad.com/mexicos_drug
_war/dto-101-the-beltran-leyva-organization.html.

76 "Mexican Drug Cartels: Update," Stratfor, May 17, 2010.

77 "4 Decapitated Bodies Hung from Bridge in Mexico" *USA Today*, August 22, 2010, http://www.usatoday.com/news/world/2010-08-22-drug-war-mexico_N.htm.

78 Stewart and Posey, "Mexico: The War with the Cartels."

79 Tim Johnson, "Rehab Clinics Turn into Killing Zones in Mexico's Drug Wars,"McLatchy News, July 22, 2010, http://www.mcclatchydc.com/2010/07/22 /97984/rehab-clinics-turn-into-killing.html.

80 Alicia Caldwell, "U.S. Official: Mexican Car Bomb Likely Used Tovex," *Washington Post*, July 19, 2010, http://www.washingtonpost.com/wp-dyn/content/article/2010 /07/19/AR2010071901027.html.

81 Foreign Military Studies Office, Latin America Security Watch, "Mexico: Special Interest," July 19, 2010. http://www.elagoradechihuahua.com/Amenazan-con-mas -coches-bomba,25606.html.

82 Hannah Stone, "New Cartel Takes Over from Familia Michoacana," insightcrime.org, March 14, 2011, http://insightcrime.org/insight-latest-news/item/671-new-cartel -announces-take-over-from-familia-michoacan.

83 Grayson, *Mexico,* 198.

84 Joseph Michael Reynolds, "From Focus on the Family to Familia Michoacana,"*July Dogs* (blog), June 2, 2009, http://julydogs.wordpress.com/2009/06/02/from-focus -on-the-family-to-la-familia-michoacana/.

85 Tim Padget, "Mexico's Meth Warriors," *Time*, June 28, 2010, http://www.time.com /time/magazine/article/0,9171,1997449,00.html.

86 Ibid.

87 "The Search for El Chayo's Body," *Borderland Beat*, December 13, 2010, http://www.borderlandbeat.com/2010/12/search-for-el-chayos-body.html.

88 "Mexico Strikes Blow to Highest Level of Feared Drug Cartel," *Borderland Beat*, December 12, 2010, http://www.borderlandbeat.com/2010/12/mexico-strikes-blow -to-highest-level-of.html.

89 "Cult-Like Gang Gains Power in Mexico's Drug Wars," Reuters, July 22, 2009, http://www.reuters.com/article/idUSN22401501.

90 Finnegan, "Silver or Lead?," 48.

91 Ioan Grillo, "Drug Dealing for Jesus: Mexico's Evangelical Narcos,"*Time*, July 19, 2009, http://www.time.com/time/world/article/0,8599,1911556,00.html.

92 Manwaring, A *"New" Dynamic*, 18.

93 Hal Brands, "Los Zetas and Mexico's Transnational Drug War," World Politics Review, December 29, 2009, http://www.worldpoliticsreview.com/articles/4866/los -zetas-and-mexicos-transnational-drug-war.

94 United States Department of Justice, *National Drug Threat Assessment 2008* (Washington, DC: National Drug Intelligence Center, 2007).

95 Manuel Roig-Franzia, "Mexican Drug Cartels Make Audacious Pitch for Recruits,"*Washington Post*, May 7, 2008, http://www.washingtonpost.com/wp-dyn /content/article/2008/05/06/AR2008050602566.html. The reference to "cup-o

-noodles" is a taunt about the basic rations that new military recruits are given when they enter basic training.

96 Lisa J. Campbell, "Los Zetas: An Operational Assessment," *Small Wars and Insurgencies* (March 2010), 67.

97 Rob Quinn, "Mexican Cartel Kills Fourth Blogger," newser.com, November 11, 2011, http://www.newser.com/story/133081/mexican-cartel-kills-4th-blogger.html.

98 Grayson, *Mexico*, 185.

99 Campbell, "Los Zetas," 73.

100 Ibid., 72.

101 Manwaring, *A "New" Dynamic*, 21.

102 "Migrants Said to Be Shot for Refusing to Become Drug Killers," msnbc.com, August 26, 2010, http://www.msnbc.msn.com/id/38867434/ns/world_news-americas/.

103 John P. Sullivan, "Police-Military Interaction in Mexico's Drug War," *Air and Space Power Journal* (October 2009), http://www.airpower.au.af.mil/apjinternational /apj-s/2009/3tri09/sullivaneng.htm.

104 Jen Phillips, "Mexico's New Super-Cartel Ups Violence in Power Play," *Mother Jones*, April 13, 2010, http://motherjones.com/mojo/2010/04/evolution-mexicos-cartel-war.

105 William Booth, "Mexican Cartels Now Using 'Tanks,'" *Washington Post*, June 7, 2011, http://www.washingtonpost.com/world/americas/mexican-cartels-now-using -tanks/2011/06/06/AGacrALH_story.html.

106 "Que quieren de nosotros?" *El Diario de Juarez*, September 20, 2010, http://www.diario .com.mx/notas.php?f=2010/09/19&id=ce557112f34b187454d7b6d117a76cb5. Translated from Spanish: "Señores de las diferentes organizaciones que se disputan la plaza de Ciudad Juárez: la pérdida de dos reporteros de esta casa editora en menos de dos años representa un quebranto irreparable para todos los que laboramos aquí y, en particular, para sus familias. Hacemos de su conocimiento que somos comunicadores, no adivinos. Portanto, como trabajadores de la información queremos que nos expliquenqué es lo que quieren de nosotros, qué es lo que pretenden que publiquemos o dejemos de publicar, para saber a qué atenernos. . . . Esta no es una rendición. Como tampoco significa que claudicamos al trabajo que hemos venido desarrollando. Se trata de una tregua para con quienes han impuesto la fuerza de su ley en esta ciudad, con tal de que respeten la vida de quienes nos dedicamos al oficio de informar."

Chapter 3. The "Battlefields": Geography of Violence and Trafficking

1 Luz Nagle, "Corruption of Politicians, Law Enforcement, and the Judiciary in Mexico and Complicity across the Border," *Small Wars and Insurgencies* (March 2010), 95.

2 Williams, "Illicit Markets, Weak States, and Violence," 329.

3 Stewart, "Mexico: The Struggle for Balance."

4 "Prevalence and Correlates of Drug Use Disorders in Mexico," *Revista Panamericana de Salud Publica*, http://www.scielosp.org/scielo.php?pid=S1020-49892006000400007 &script=sci_arttext.

5 Saul Cohen, *Geography and Politics in a Divided World* (London: Methuen, 1964), 24.

6 Ken Ellingwood, "Why Mexico Is Not the New Colombia When It Comes to Drug Cartels," *Los Angeles Times*, September 25, 2010, http://www.latimes.com /news/nationworld/world/la-fg-mexico-colombia-20100926,0,2434157.story.

7 "Organized Crime in Mexico," Stratfor.

8 Ibid.

9 "Killings Up Nearly 50% in Mexican Border City," *Latin American Herald Tribune*, October 14, 2010, http://www.laht.com/article.asp?ArticleId=361676&CategoryId =14091.

10 "Factbox: Worst Attacks in Mexico's Drug War," *Borderland Beat*, August 20, 2010.

11 "Kingpin's Cartel Winning Mexican Drug War," Fox News, April 9, 2010, http://www .foxnews.com/world/2010/04/09/ap-kingpins-cartel-winning-mexican-drug-war/.

12 Antonio Villegas, "Drug Gangs Escalate Attacks on Mexican Army," msnbc.com, April 1, 2010.

13 "New Border War Erupts with Mexico Cartel Rift," msnbc.com, March 13, 2010, http://www.msnbc.msn.com/id/36136926/ns/world_news-americas/.

14 "Organized Crime in Mexico."

15 Varese, *The Russian Mafia*, 187.

16 Ibid., 187–88.

17 Grayson, *Mexico*, 198.

18 Finnegan, "Silver or Lead?," 46.

19 David Danelo, "The Many Faces of Mexico," *Orbis* (Winter 2011), 175.

20 Mica Rosenberg, "Violence Erupts in Mexico's Drugs Heartland," Reuters, May 20, 2008, http://www.reuters.com/article/idUSN2056518720080520.

21 Ibid.

22 Bob Killebrew and Jennifer Bernal, *Crime Wars* (Center for a New American Security, September 2010), 20.

23 George Grayson, "La Familia: Another Deadly Syndicate," Foreign Policy Research Institute, February 2009, http://www.fpri.org/enotes/200901.grayson.lafamilia.html.

24 "Thursday's Attacks: Ciudad Juarez, Mexico City, Jalisco," *Borderland Beat,* October 29, 2010, http://www.borderlandbeat.com/2010/10/thursdays-attacks-ciudad -juarez-mexico.html.

25 Ibid.

26 Killebrew and Bernal, *Crime Wars*, 17.

27 Finnegan, "Silver or Lead?," 46.

28 William Booth and Nick Miroff, "Threat Increases as Mexican Cartels Move across the Border," *Buenos Aires Herald*, October 30, 2010, http://www.buenosairesherald.com/PrintedEdition/View/49012.

29 Nicholas Casey, "Mexico under Seige," *Wall Street Journal*, August 19, 2010, http://online .wsj.com/article/SB10001424052748704557704575437762646209270.html.

30 Robin Emmott, "Mexican Cartels Break Open New Front in Drugs War," Reuters, May 20, 2009, http://www.reuters.com/article/idUSN1140493820090520.

31 Ibid.

32 Diego Valle-Jones, blog.diegovalle.net.

33 Karl Penhaul, "Brave Few Break Mexico Drug War's Code of Silence," CNN, June 18, 2010, http://articles.cnn.com/2010-06-18/world/mexico.drug.war_1_cartels -drug-war-municipal-police?_s=PM:WORLD.

34 Nicholas Casey and Jose de Cordoba, "Northern Mexico's State of Anarchy," *Wall Street Journal*, November 20–21, 2010.

35 "Una Cruz de Pesa," *Borderland Beat*, November 5, 2010, http://www.borderlandbeat .com/2010/11/mexicos-2010-drug-war-stats-10000.html.

36 Killebrew and Bernal, *Crime Wars*, 8.

Chapter 4. The Spread: The Effects on the United States

1 Alberto Melis, "Foreword: A View from the Borderlands," *Small Wars and Insurgencies* (March 2010), 3.

2 Ray Walser, "Mexico, Drug Cartels, and the Merida Initiative," *Heritage Foundation Backgrounder*, July 23, 2008, 2.

3 Phil Williams, "Transnational Criminal Organizations and International Security," in *In Athena's Camp*, eds. John Arquilla and David Ronfeldt (Santa Monica, CA: Rand Corporation, 1997), 331.

4 Stratfor, *Mexico in Crisis: Lost Borders and the Struggle for Regional Status* (Austin, TX: Stratfor, 2009), 23–24.

5 Joseph M. Arabit, "Violence along the Southwest Border" (statement before the House Appropriations Committee, Subcommittee on Commerce, Justice, Science, and Related Agencies, March 24, 2009), http://www.usdoj.gov/dea/speeches/s032409.pdf.

6 Kristin Finklea, William Krouse, and Marc Rosenblum, *Southwest Border Violence: Issues in Identifying and Measuring Spillover Violence* (Washington, DC: Congressional Research Service, August 25, 2010), 24.

7 This is a broader definition of the DEA's definition of spillover violence, which specifically mentions violence but excludes trafficker-on-trafficker violence. See Arabit, "Violence along the Southwest Border," 5.

8 Michael Hayes (Special Agent, U.S. Border Patrol), interview, June 12, 2010.

9 "On the Southwest Border: Public Corruption," *Federal Bureau of Investigation News*, August 9, 2010, http://www.fbi.gov/news/stories/2010/august/southwest -border2/border-corruption.

10 "Mexican Drug Gangs Able to Corrupt Border Patrol," *Pittsburgh Tribune-Review*, March 12, 2010, http://www.pittsburghlive.com/x/pittsburghtrib/news/s_671257.html.

11 Sebastian Rotella, "Former U.S. Anti-Drug Official Arrest 'A Complete Shock,'" *Los Angeles Times*, September 17, 2009, http://articles.latimes.com/2009/sep/17 /nation/na-drug-charges17.

12 Randal Archibold, "Hired by Customs, but Working for Mexican Cartels," *New York Times*, December 17, 2009, http://www.nytimes.com/2009/12/18/us/18corrupt.html ?pagewanted=all.

13 Paul Weber, "U.S. Border Patrol Agents in 'Firefight' with Mexican Gang," ABC News, September 13, 2010, http://abcnews.go.com/US/wirestory?id=11627914&page=2.

14 National Drug Intelligence Center, *Arizona: High-Intensity Drug Trafficking Area, Drug Market Analysis 2009* (March 2009), 13.

15 United States Agency for International Development, *Central America and Mexico Gang Assessment* (April 2006), 9.

16 Jonathan Clark, "Drug Cartel Issues Threat to Off-Duty Nogales Police Officers," *Nogales International*, June 18, 2010, http://www.nogalesinternational.com/articles /2010/06/18/news/breaking_news/doc4c1c0aa77f1de517562478.txt.

17 "Border Patrol Agent Killed in Southern Arizona," msnbc.com, December 15, 2010, http://www.msnbc.msn.com/id/40678058/ns/us_news-crime_and_courts/.

18 Jerry Seper, "Mexican Military Incursions Reported," *Washington Times*, January 17, 2006, 1. It must be noted that the Mexican government denies these incursions and believes that these incursions are by Los Zetas who often wear military uniforms and use military-style tactics and military vehicles.

19 "Mexican Military Incursion in Texas," Judicial Watch, March 12, 2010, http://www.judicialwatch.org/blog/2010/mar/mexican-military-incursion-texas.

20 Diana Washington Valdez and Daniel Borunda, "Mexican Drone Crashes in Backyard of El Paso Home," *El Paso Times*, December 17, 2010, http://www.elpasotimes.com /ci_16875462.

21 Daniel Wood, "Robert Krentz Killing Stokes Fears of Rampant Illegal Immigration," *Christian Science Monitor*, March 31, 2010, http://www.csmonitor.com/USA/2010 /0331/Robert-Krentz-killing-stokes-fears-of-rampant-illegal-immigration. The author also interviewed the neighbors of Robert Krentz, who tracked his killer south to the Mexican border. The killer was likely returning to Mexico after completing his smuggling when he encountered Robert Krentz. The killer has not been captured, and the exact nature of his business or what occurred is pieced together with a good deal of circumstantial evidence.

22 William Booth, "Mexican Pirates Attack Texas Fishermen on Falcon Lake, Which Straddles Border," *Washington Post*, May 30, 2010.

23 Ibid.

24 Patrik Jonnson, "Mistaken Identity Theory Gains Traction in Falcon Lake 'Pirate' Attack," *Christian Science Monitor*, October 15, 2010, http://www.csmonitor.com/USA/2010 /1015/Mistaken-identity-theory-gains-traction-in-Falcon-Lake-pirate-attack.

25 Patrik Jonnson, "Falcon Lake 'Pirate' Murder: Is Beheading 'Message to the Americans'?" *Christian Science Monitor*, October 13, 2010, http://www.csmonitor.com /USA/2010/1013/Falcon-Lake-pirate-murder-Is-beheading-message-to-the-Americans.

26 Booth, "Mexican Pirates Attack."

27 United States Fish and Wildlife Service, *Closure of Refuge Lands Adjacent to Border: Buenos Aires National Wildlife Refuge*, http://www.fws.gov/southwest/refuges/arizona/buenosaires/PDFs/Closure.pdf.

28 Dan Simon, "Mexican Cartels Running Pot Farms in U.S. National Forest," CNN, August 8, 2008, http://articles.cnn.com/2008-08-08/justice/pot.eradication_1_marijuana-plants-drug-cartels-pot-production?_s=PM:CRIME.

29 Jose Millman, "Mexican Pot Gangs Infiltrate Indian Reservations in the U.S.," *Wall Street Journal*, November 5, 2009, http://online.wsj.com/article/SB125736987377028727.html.

30 "Mexican Pot Gangs Pollute National Parks," CBS News, October 11, 2008, http://www.cbsnews.com/stories/2008/10/11/national/main4515320.shtml?tag=topHome;topStories.

31 Millman, "Mexican Pot Gangs Infiltrate Indian Reservations in the U.S."

32 Kimberley Dvorak, "Los Zetas Drug Cartel Seizes 2 U.S. Ranches in Texas," *San Diego Examiner*, July 24, 2010, http://www.examiner.com/county-political-buzz-in-san-diego/los-zetas-drug-cartel-seizes-2-u-s-ranches-texas.

33 National Drug Intelligence Center, *National Drug Threat Assessment 2010*, http://www.justice.gov/ndic/pubs38/38661/movement.htm#Flow.

34 Ibid.

35 Sergio Chapa, "ICE Agents Bust Armed Convoy in San Benito," KGBT News Channel 4, November 18, 2010, http://www.valleycentral.com/news/story.aspx?id=542803.

36 National Drug Intelligence Center, *National Drug Threat Assessment 2009*, 45.

37 Williams, "Transnational Criminal Organizations," 329.

38 Ibid.

39 National Drug Intelligence Center, *Arizona: High-Intensity Drug Trafficking Area*, 14.

40 Alicia Caldwell, "Mexican Drug Violence Spills Over into U.S.," Huffingtonpost.com, February 11, 2009, http://www.huffingtonpost.com/2009/02/09/mexican-drug-violence-spi_n_165422.html.

41 Bunker, Campbell, and Bunker, "Torture, Beheadings, and Narcocultos," 150, 160; and Joel Waldman, "Police: Chandler, AZ Beheading Possible Cartel Hit," KGUN9 News, October 30, 2010, http://www.kgun9.com/Global/story.asp?S=13414677.

42 Amanda Lee Myers, "Cops: Arizona Beheading Linked to Mexican Cartel," msnbc.com, March 3, 2011, http://www.msnbc.msn.com/id/41883795/ns/us_news-crime_and_courts/t/cops-ariz-beheading-linked-mexican-cartel/.

43 Laurie Freeman, *State of Siege: Drug-Related Violence and Corruption in Mexico*, Washington Office on Latin America Special Report, June 2006, 10.

44 Robert Killebrew, "A New Threat: The Crossover of Urban Gang Warfare and Terrorism," *National Strategy Forum Review* (Fall 2008), 5.

45 Stratfor, *Mexico in Crisis*, 61.

46 "Convicted Houston Gun Trafficker for Zeta Cartel Sentenced to Three Years," *Borderland Beat*, January 5, 2011, http://www.borderlandbeat.com/2011/01/convicted-houston-gun-trafficker-for.html.

47 James C. McKinley Jr., "U.S. Is Arms Bazaar for Mexican Cartels," *New York Times*, February 25, 2009, http://www.nytimes.com/2009/02/26/us/26borders.html.

48 Stratfor, *Mexico in Crisis*, 63.

49 "Soldier Accused of Being Hit Man for Cartel," CNN, August 12, 2009, http://www.cnn.com/2009/CRIME/08/11/texas.soldier.arrested/index.html?eref=rss_latest.

50 U.S. Department of Justice, National Gang Intelligence Center, *National Gang Threat Assessment 2009*, http://www.justice.gov/ndic/pubs32/32146/military.htm.

51 "'I Slit Their Throats,' Accused Teen Hit Man Says," CNN, December 5, 2010, http://www.cnn.com/2010/WORLD/americas/12/05/mexico.teen.hit.man/index.html.

52 James C. McKinley Jr., "Mexican Cartels Lure American Teens as Killers," *New York Times*, June 23, 2009, http://www.nytimes.com/2009/06/23/us/23killers.html.

53 Ibid.

54 Michael Smith, "Banks Financing Mexican Gangs Admitted in Wells Fargo Deal," *Bloomberg News*, June 29, 2010, http://www.bloomberg.com/news/2010-06-29/banks-financing-mexico-s-drug-cartels-admitted-in-wells-fargo-s-u-s-deal.html.

55 Brady McCombs, "U.S. Seizing Drug Money but Cartels Have Plenty More," *Arizona Daily Star*, March 7, 2010, http://azstarnet.com/news/local/govt-and-politics/02b2696c-2401-58fc-9f59-3286674b8a6d.html.

56 Janice Kephart, "Enhancing DHS' Efforts to Disrupt Alien Smuggling across the Border" (testimony before House Committee on Homeland Security, Subcommittee on Border, Maritime, and Global Counterterrorism, July 22, 2010), http://www.cis.org/node/2109.

57 William Booth and Nick Miroff, "Traffickers along U.S.-Mexico Border Turn to Disguises," *Washington Post*, August 31, 2010.

58 William Booth, "Drug Smugglers along Border Use Innocent Disguises," *Seattle Times*, September 18, 2010, http://seattletimes.nwsource.com/html/nationworld/2012929858_borderdrugs19.html.

59 Robert Bunker, "Strategic Threat: Narcs and Narcotics Overview," 18.

60 National Drug Intelligence Center, *National Drug Threat Assessment 2008*, http://www.justice.gov/ndic/pubs25/25921/border.htm.

61 Killebrew, "A New Threat," 12.

62 William Booth, "U.S. Agents to Fight Drug Cartels in Mexico," msnbc.com, February 24, 2010, http://msnbc.msn.com/id/35556681/ns/world_news-washington_post/.

63 "Over 200,000 Leave Mexico Border City," *Latin America Herald Tribune*, October 14, 2010, http://www.laht.com/article.asp?ArticleId=367604&CategoryId=14091.

64 Jason Beaubien, "In Just One Year, A Mexican City Turns Violent," National Public Radio, October 16, 2010, http://www.npr.org/templates/story/story.php?storyId=130592600.

65 "Threats from Narcos Force Mayors to Live in U.S.," *Borderland Beat*, September 27, 2010, http://www.borderlandbeat.com/2010/09/threats-from-narcos-force-mexican.html.

66 Ibid.

67 Luhnow and de Cordoba, "The Perilous State of Mexico."

68 Ibid.

69 "Porque se fue Alejandro Junco," *Reporte Indigo*, www.reporteindigo.com, September 12, 2008, http://octavioislas.wordpress.com/2008/09/13/1732-mexico-reporte-indigo-12-de-septiembre-de-2008-nuevo-periodismo-digital-en-mexico/.

70 Jacqui Goddard, "Interpol Agent Passed Information to the Beltran-Leyva Cartel in Mexico," *Times of London*, October 28, 2008, http://www.timesonline.co.uk/tol/news/world/us_and_americas/article5026787.ece.

71 "Mexican Drug Cartels: An Update," Stratfor.

72 "Fifth American Killed in Mexican Border City in Past Week," msnbc.com, November 3, 2010, http://www.msnbc.msn.com/id/39998294/ns/world_news-americas.

73 Richard Coraggio (Special Agent, Immigration and Customs Enforcement, Criminal Division), New York City, interview, November 19, 2008.

74 Casey, "Mexico under Seige."

75 "A One-Two Punch," *The Economist*, May 29, 2010, 40.

76 Nicholas Casey and James Hagerty, "Companies Shun Violent Mexico," *Wall Street Journal*, December 17, 2010, http://online.wsj.com/article/SB10001424052748703395204576023811983098994.html?mod=WSJ_hp_MIDDLENexttoWhatsNewsTop.

77 Mica Rosenberg, "Mexican Violence Hits U.S. 'Salad Bowl,'" msnbc.com, December 22, 2010, http://www.msnbc.msn.com/id/40772711/ns/business-us_business/.

78 Stewart, "Mexico: The Struggle for Balance."

79 Booth, "U.S. Agents to Fight Drug Cartels in Mexico."

80 Casey and de Codoba, "Northern Mexico's State of Anarchy."

81 "Thousands of Ranches Abandoned in Tamaulipas Due to Violence," *Borderland Beat*, November 27, 2010, http://www.borderlandbeat.com/2010/11/thousands-of-ranches-abandoned-in.html.

82 John Arquilla and David Ronfeldt, eds., *Networks and Netwars* (Santa Monica, CA: Rand, 2001), 78.

83 "Mexican Drug Cartels Expanding Influence to 47 Nations," Associated Press, July 21, 2009.

84 Thomas Bruneau, "The Maras and National Security in Central America," *Strategic Insights* (May 2005), 5.

85 Hal Brands, *Crime, Violence, and the Crisis in Guatemala* (Carlisle Barracks, PA: Strategic Studies Institute, 2010), 2.

86 Lindsay Stewart and Jennifer Griffin, "America's Third War: U.S. Secretly Trains Guatemalan Forces," Fox News, December 14, 2010, http://www.foxnews.com /us/2010/12/14/americas-war-secretly-trains-guatemalan-forces/.

87 Hal Brands, *Crime, Violence, and the Crisis in Guatemala* (Carlisle Barracks, PA: Strategic Studies Institute, 2010), 14.

88 Adam Elkus, "Gangs, Terrorists, and Trade," *Foreign Policy in Focus*, April 12, 2007, http://www.fpif.org/articles/gangs_terrorists_and_trade.

89 "Gang Linked to Honduras Massacre," BBC News, December 24, 2004, http://news.bbc.co.uk/2/hi/americas/4124133.stm.

90 Hannah Stone, "FARC-Mexican Cartel Middlemen Captured in Colombia," *Colombia Reports*, August 31, 2010, http://colombiareports.com/colombia-news /news/11604-farc-mexican-cartel-middlemen-captured-in-colombia.html.

91 "Colombia Rebels Linked to Mexican Drug Cartels," *New York Times*, October 7, 2008, http://www.nytimes.com/2008/10/08/world/americas/08mexico.html?_r=2.

92 Stratfor, *Mexico in Crisis*, 197.

93 Francisco Gomez, "Indagan Red De Mafia Japonesa en Mexico," *El Universal*, December 5, 2010, http://www.eluniversal.com.mx/nacion/182273.html.

94 Arthur Brice, "Latin American Drug Cartels Find Home in West Africa," CNN, September 21, 2009, http://articles.cnn.com/2009-09-21/world/africa.drug.cartels _1_drug-cartels-european-market-cocaine?_s=PM:WORLD.

95 Phillip Sherwell, "Cocaine, Kidnapping, and the Al Qaeda Cash Squeeze," *Sunday Telegraph*, March 6, 2010, http://www.telegraph.co.uk/news/worldnews /africaandindianocean/mali/7386278/Cocaine-kidnapping-and-the-Al-Qaeda-cash -squeeze.html; Aida Alami, "Morocco Battles Al Qaeda in the Islamic Maghreb," *Global Post*, November 2, 2010, http://www.globalpost.com/dispatch/morocco /101101/morocco-battles-al-qaeda-the-islamic-maghreb.

96 Beith, "Are Mexico's Drug Cartels Terrorist Groups?"

97 Ibid.

98 Phil Williams, "Organizing Transnational Crime," in *Combating Transnational Crime*, ed. Phil Williams and Dimitri Vlassis (Portland, OR: Frank Cass, 2001), 61.

99 Stratfor, *Mexico in Crisis*, 177.

100 Stewart and Griffin, "America's Third War: U.S. Secretly Trains Guatemalan Forces."

101 Tim Palmer, "Mexican Drug Cartel Infiltrates Australia," Australian Broadcasting Corporation, September 15, 2010, http://www.sbs.com.au/news/article/1407306 /latest-from-wire/.

102 Doris Gomora, "Carteles Mexicanos Compran Droga en Afghanistan, Alertan," *El Universal*, January 4, 2011, http://www.eluniversal.com.mx/notas/734815.html.

103 Anthony Placido and Kevin Perkins, "Drug Trafficking Violence in Mexico: Implications for the United States" (statement before the Senate Caucus on International Narcotics Control, United States Senate, May 5, 2010), 6, http://www.justice.gov/dea/speeches/100505_inc.pdf.

104 James McKinley Jr., "Suspect in Juarez Says Killers Pursued Jail Guard," *New York Times*, March 31, 2010, http://www.nytimes.com/2010/04/01/world/americas/01mexico.html.

105 Lourdes Medrano, "Border Patrol Agent Killed: Are Smugglers Becoming More Daring?" *Christian Science Monitor*, December 15, 2010, http://www.csmonitor.com /USA/2010/1215/Border-patrol-agent-killed-Are-smugglers-becoming-more-daring.

Chapter 5. The "Guardians": Law Enforcement and the Judiciary

1 Freeman, *State of Siege*, 6.

2 David Bayley, and Robert Perito, *The Police in War* (Boulder, CO: Lynne Rienner, 2010), 76.

3 When U.S. Secretary of State Hillary Clinton compared the situation in Mexico to an insurgency "more like Colombia looked twenty years ago," President Obama quickly distanced the U.S. government from the comparison while the Mexican government quickly rejected it. See Tom Peter, "Mexico Denies Hillary Clinton's 'Insurgency' Comparison," *Christian Science Monitor*, September 9, 2010, http://www.csmonitor.com/World/terrorism-security/2010/0909/Mexico-denies -Hillary-Clinton-s-insurgency-comparison. After the first car bomb was used in Mexico, the Mexican attorney general, Arturo Chavez, refused to declare it an act of terrorism or "narco-terrorism." See Maggie Ybarra and Daniel Borunda, "Mexico Attorney General: Juarez Explosion Not 'Narco-Terrorism,'" *El Paso Times*, July 16, 2010, http://www.elpasotimes.com/ci_15531121.

4 Kenney, *From Pablo to Osama*, 80–81.

5 Ibid., 107.

6 Ibid., 105.

7 Ibid., 106.

8 Nagle, "Corruption of Politicians, Law Enforcement, and the Judiciary in Mexico and Complicity across the Border," 96.

9 "Under the Volcano," *The Economist*, October 16, 2010, 30.

10 Diego Cevallos, "Police Caught between Low Wages, Threats, and Bribes," *International Press Service News*, June 7, 2009, http://ipsnews.net/news.asp?idnews=38075.

11 Transparency International, *Global Corruption Report 2007*, 15.

12 United Nations Special Rapporteur, *Independence of Judges and Lawyers: Report on the Mission to Mexico*, January 24, 2002, 18.

13 Jose Fernandez Menendez, *Mexico: The Traffickers' Judges, Global Corruption Report 2007*, Transparency International.

14 David Shirk, "Justice Reform in Mexico, Working Paper Series on U.S.-Mexico Security Cooperation" (Transborder Institute: University of San Diego, April 2010), 9–10.

15 Sara Miller Llana, "Setbacks in Mexico's War on Corruption," *Christian Science Monitor*, December 30, 2008, http://www.csmonitor.com/World/Americas/2008/1230/p06s02-woam.html.

16 Placido and Perkins, "Drug Trafficking Violence in Mexico," 7.

17 T. Kellne and F. Pipitone, *Inside Mexico's Drug War* (New York: World Policy Institute, 2010).

18 "Under the Volcano," 30.

19 Ibid.

20 Llana, "Setbacks in Mexico's War on Corruption."

21 Placido and Perkins, "Drug Trafficking Violence in Mexico," 7.

22 Randal Archibald, "Mexican Prosecutors Train in U.S. for Changes in their Legal System," *New York Times*, April 24, 2009, http://www.nytimes.com/2009/04/25/us/25prosecute.html.

23 Stratfor, *Mexico in Crisis*, 149.

24 Jason Beaubien, "Saint or Sinner?," National Public Radio, April 13, 2009, http://www.npr.org/templates/story/story.php?storyId=102928118.

25 Tracy Wilkinson and Ken Ellingwood, "Mexico's Army Failures Hamper Drug War," *Los Angeles Times*, December 29, 2010, http://articles.latimes.com/2010/dec/29/world/la-fg-mexico-army-20101230.

26 "Mexico Drug Killings Peak Amid Offensive," *USA Today*, January 13, 2011.

27 Danelo, "The Many Faces of Mexico," 165.

28 Ibid., 172.

29 "Falling Kingpins, Rising Violence," *The Economist*, December 18, 2010, 56.

30 Olivia Torres, "7 Killed at Park in Besieged Mexican Border City," msnbc.com, January 24, 2011, http://www.msnbc.msn.com/id/41241921/ns/world_news-americas/.

31 Ibid.

32 Danelo, "The Many Faces of Mexico," 173.

33 "Mexico Aims to Protect Reporters from Cartel Violence," msnbc.com, September 23, 2010, http://www.msnbc.msn.com/id/39318581/ns/world_news-americas/.

34 Miroff, "Mexico Hopes $270 Million in Social Spending Will Help End Juarez Drug Violence."

35 Henry Cuellar, "Five Perspectives on the Mérida Initiative," American Enterprise Institute, March 2008, 2.

36 Claire Seelke and Kristin Finklea, *U.S.-Mexican Security Cooperation: The Mérida Initiative and Beyond* (Washington, DC: Congressional Research Service, 2010).

37 *Status of Funds for the Mérida Initiative* (Government Accountability Office, December 3, 2009), 5.

38 White House Office of the Press Secretary, "Declaration by the Government of the United States of America and the Government of the United Mexican States Concerning Twenty-First Century Border Management," press release, May 19, 2010.

39 Viola Gienger, "Mexico, U.S. Expand Drug War beyond Military to Social Efforts," *Bloomberg Business Week*, March 24, 2010, http://www.businessweek.com/news/2010-03-24/mexico-u-s-expand-drug-war-beyond-military-to-social-efforts.html.

40 Seelke and Finklea, *U.S.-Mexican Security Cooperation*, 26.

41 Ibid., 27.

42 Placido and Perkins, "Drug Trafficking Violence in Mexico," 9.

43 Grayson, *Mexico,* 242.

44 *Specially Designated Nationals List,* U.S. Department of the Treasury, Resource Center, http://www.treasury.gov/resource-center/sanctions/SDN-List/Pages/default.aspx.

45 Placido and Perkins, "Drug Trafficking Violence in Mexico," 31.

46 Carrie Johnson, "Holder Takes the Heat over 'Fast and Furious' Scandal," National Public Radio, October 6, 2011, http://www.npr.org/2011/10/06/141124685 /holder-takes-heat-over-fast-and-furious-scandal.

47 Mary Beth Sheridan, "Military Broadens U.S. Push to Help Mexico Battle Drug Cartels," *Washington Post,* November 10, 2010.

48 Ibid.

49 Susan Ginsburg, *Security Human Mobility in an Age of Risk* (Washington, DC: Migration Policy Institute, 2010), 7.

50 Peter Andreas, *Border Games* (Ithaca, NY: Cornell University Press, 2009), 4.

51 Payan, *The Three U.S.-Mexico Border Wars,* 20.

52 Booth, "U.S. Agents to Fight Drug Cartels in Mexico."

53 U.S. Department of State, "Office for the Mérida Initiative Opens in Mexico City," press release, August 31, 2010, http://www.america.gov/st/texttrans-english/2010 /August/20100901111635su0.0598653.html#ixzz19nO0RXvr.

54 Andreas, *Border Games,* 144–45.

55 Kenney, *From Pablo to Osama,* 120.

56 "Mexican Government Says Security Strategy Has Been a Success," *Borderland Beat,* January 4, 2011, http://www.borderlandbeat.com/2011/01/mexican-government -says-security.html.

57 "Falling Kingpins, Rising Violence," *The Economist,* December 18, 2010.

58 Seelke and Finklea, *U.S.-Mexican Security Cooperation,* 11.

59 Interview with Border Patrol, San Diego Sector, June 12, 2010.

Chapter 6. The Harbingers: Possible Outcomes

1 In reading multiple versions of Sun Tzu's *Art of War,* I have not found this quote in any. The quote, however, continues to be ascribed to him.

2 Phillip Le Billon, "The Political Ecology of War: Natural Resources and Armed Conflict," *Political Geography* (June 2001); and Michael L. Ross, "Oil, Drugs, and Diamonds: The Varying Roles of Natural Resources in Civil War," in *The Political Economy of Armed Conflict,* eds. Karen Ballentine and Jake Sherman (Boulder, CO: Lynne Rienner, 2003).

3 Indra de Soysa, "The Resource Curse: Are Civil Wars Driven by Rapacity or Paucity?" in *Greed and Grievance: Economic Agendas in Civil Wars,* eds. Mats Berdal and David

Malone (Boulder, CO: Lynne Rienner, 2000); David Kean, "Incentives and Disincentives for Violence" in *Greed and Grievance*, ed. Berdal and Malone.

4 "Roman Catholics Around the World," BBC News, April 1, 2005, http://news.bbc.co.uk/2/hi/4243727.stm.

5 David Bayley, *Changing the Guard* (New York: Oxford University Press, 2006).

6 Alexandra Olson, "Amid Drug War, Mexico Less Deadly than a Decade Ago," *El Paso Times*, February 7, 2010, http://www.elpasotimes.com/texas/ci_14353710.

7 Grim, *This Is Your Country on Drugs*, 118.

8 "The Democratic Routine," *The Economist*, December 4, 2010, 51.

9 Selee, Shirk, and Olson, "Five Myths."

10 United Nations Office on Drugs and Crime, "The Threat of Narco Trafficking in the Americas," October 2008, 35.

11 Sergio Flores and Mark Walsh, "13 Mexican Troops Charged with Transporting Drugs," Associated Press, March 4, 2010; and Jose de Cordoba and David Luhnow, "Mexican Army Officers Detained for Cartel Payments," *Wall Street Journal*, June 15, 2009, http://online.wsj.com/article/SB124510705768916735.html.

12 Steve Fainaru and William Booth, "Mexico Using Torture to Battle Drug Trafficker, Rights Groups Say," *Washington Post*, July 9, 2009, http://www.washingtonpost.com/wp-dyn/content/article/2009/07/08/AR2009070804197.html.

13 Nacha Cattan, "UN Questions Mexican Army's Role in Drug War," *Christian Science Monitor*, April 1, 2011, http://www.csmonitor.com/World/Americas/2011/0401/UN-questions-Mexican-Army-s-role-in-drug-war.

14 Ibid.

15 Peter Lupsha, "Transnational Organized Crime Versus the State," *Transnational Organized Crime* (Spring 1996), 27.

16 Robert J. Bunker and John P. Sullivan, "Cartel Evolution Revisited: Third Phase Cartel Potentials and Alternative Futures in Mexico," *Small Wars and Insurgencies* (March 2010), 48.

17 Ibid.

18 United States Joint Forces Command, *Joint Operating Environment 2008* (November 25, 2008), 36.

19 Patrick Corcoran, "Release of Mexico Murder Stats Reveals Shifting Landscape," insightcrime.org, October 23, 2011, http://insightcrime.org/insight-latest-news/item/1744-release-of-mexico-government-info-reveals-shifting-landscape.

20 Brian Jenkins, "Mexico: Failing State?" *National Journal*, March 23, 2009, http://security.nationaljournal.com/2009/03/mexico-failing-state.php.

21 Manuel Perez-Rocha, "Mexico: Neither a Failed State nor Model," Institute for Policy Studies, February 23, 2009, http://www.ips-dc.org/articles/mexico_neither_a_failed_state_nor_a_model.

22 NationMaster, "Crime Statistics," nationmaster.com, 2008, http://www.nationmaster.com/red/pie/cri_tot_cri-crime-total-crimes.

23 Juan Nava, "Mexico: Failing State or Emerging Democracy?" *Military Review* (March–April 2011), 39.

24 Corcoran, "Release of Mexico Murder Stats."

25 Daniel Hernandez, "Mexico Expats Warned on Travel Home," *Los Angeles Times*, November 24, 2010.

26 William Lajeunesse, "Uncovering Border Tunnels," Fox News, November 23, 2010, http://www.foxnews.com/us/2010/11/23/americas-war-smuggling-tunnels/.

27 Robert Bonner, "New Cocaine Cowboys," *Foreign Affairs* (July/August 2010).

28 Grayson, *Mexico*, 258.

29 "Saddling Up for the Trail to Los Pinos," *The Economist*, January 29, 2011, 34.

30 Ibid.

31 Sara Miller Llana, "Mexico's La Familia Cartel to Government: We'll Disband If You Protect Citizens," *Christian Science Monitor*, November 11, 2010, http://www.csmonitor.com/World/Global-News/2010/1111/Mexico-s-La-Familia -cartel-to-government-We-ll-disband-if-you-protect-citizens.

32 "Falling Kingpins," 56.

33 Lupsha, "Transnational Organized Crime Versus the State," 32.

34 Bunker and Sullivan, "Cartel Evolution Revisited," 49.

35 Diego Enrique Osorno, "Vigilante Groups Appear in Five Mexican States," *El Milenio*, January 26, 2009, http://narcosphere.narconews.com/notebook/kristin-bricker /2009/01/vigilante-groups-appear-five-mexican-states.

36 Ibid.

37 David Luhnow and Jose de Cordoba, "The Perilous State of Mexico," *Wall Street Journal*, February 21, 2009, http://online.wsj.com/article/SB123518102536038463.html.

38 Bunker, Campbell, and Bunker, "Torture, Beheadings, and Narcocultos," 150.

39 David Luhnow, "Elite Flee Drug War in Mexico's No. 3 City," *Wall Street Journal*, September 10, 2010, http://online.wsj.com/article /SB10001424052748704644404575482573438556534.html

40 Ibid.

41 Casey and Hagerty, "Companies Shun Violent Mexico."

42 Stewart, "Mexico: The Struggle for Balance."

43 David Agren, "Oil: The Mexican Cartels' Other Deadly Business," *Toronto Globe and Mail*, December 21, 2010, http://www.theglobeandmail.com/news/world /americas/oil-the-mexican-cartels-other-deadly-business/article1845378/.

44 Laurence Iliff and Alfredo Corchado, "Drug Violence Has Moved into Mexico City," *Dallas Morning News*, February 8, 2008, http://www.dallasnews.com /sharedcontent/dws/news/texassouthwest/stories/DN- capital_08int.ART.North.Edition1.45119ad.html.

45 Stratfor, *Mexico in Crisis*.

46 "Drug Violence Creeps into Mexico City," msnbc.com, December 27, 2011, http://www
    .msnbc.msn.com/id/45795224/ns/world_news-americas/#.TvovfmAW8bU.

47 Nate Freier, *Known Unknowns: Strategic Shocks in Defense Strategy Development*
    (Carlisle Barracks, PA: Strategic Studies Institute, 2008), 11–15.

48 Nacha Cattan, "Fed Up with Plague of Kidnappings, Mexicans Turn to Mob
    Justice," *Christian Science Monitor*, September 22, 2010, http://www.csmonitor.com/
    World/Americas/2010/0922/Fed-up-with-plague-of-kidnappings-Mexicans-turn
    -to-mob-justice.

49 "Threats from Narcos Force Mayors to Live in U.S."

50 Stratfor, *Mexico in Crisis*, 96.

Chapter 7: Finding the End: Recommendations and Responses

1 Entous and Hodge, "U.S. Sees Heightened Threat in Mexico."

2 Ted Galen Carpenter, "Mexico Is Becoming the Next Colombia," CATO Institute
   Foreign Policy Briefing no. 87, November 15, 2005.

3 Independent Commission on Policing in Northern Ireland, *A New Beginning:
   Policing in Northern Ireland* (Belfast: Her Majesty's Stationery Office, 1999), 18.

4 Bayley and Perito, *The Police in War*, 75.

5 Bayley, *Changing the Guard*, 75.

6 Alan Wright, *Organised Crime* (Cullompton, UK: Willan, 2006), 185.

7 Robert MacCoun and Peter Reuter, *Drug War Heresies* (Cambridge, UK: Cambridge
   University Press, 2001), 8.

8 See Allan Brandt, *The Cigarette Century* (New York: Basic Books, 2007), 449–65.

9 Beau Kilmer, Jonathan P. Caulkins, Brittany M. Bond, and Peter H. Reuter, "Reducing
   Drug Trafficking Revenues and Violence in Mexico," Rand Corporation, 2010, 57.

10 Ibid. "Expressive violence is force used for personal and emotional reasons. Instrumental
   violence is force for the purposes of accomplishing a functional goal. It is a common
   distinction in criminology."

11 Varese, *The Russian Mafia*, 190.

12 Mica Rosenberg, "Drug Gangs Clash with Dogged Miners in Mexico," Reuters,
   April 14, 2010, http://www.reuters.com/article/2011/04/14/us-mexico-drugs
   -mining-idUSTRE73D5FH20110414.

13 Ronan Graham, "Are Mexican Drug Gangs Drafting Hackers?" insightcrime.org,
   July 17, 2011, http://insightcrime.org/insight-latest-news/item/1251-are-mexico
   -drug-gangs-drafting-hackers.

14 John Sullivan, "Counter-Supply and Counter-Violence Approaches to Narcotics
   Trafficking," *Small Wars and Insurgencies* (March 2010), 180.

15 Beith, "Are Mexico's Drug Cartels Terrorist Groups?"

16 Many thanks to Nick Iorio for finding this information on Mexican policing.

17 Lauren Villagran and Olivia Torres, "Ciudad Juarez 'Safe Corridors' Plagued by Killings," msnbc.com, March 13, 2011, http://www.msnbc.msn.com/id/42062201/ns/world_news-americas/.

18 Spencer Hsu and Mary Beth Sheridan, "Anti-Drug Effort at U.S. Border Readied," *Washington Post*, March 22, 2009.

19 Fisman and Miguel, *Economic Gangsters*, 190.

20 O'Neill, "The Real War in Mexico," 66.

21 "Under the Volcano," 31.

22 Glenn Greenwald, "Drug Decriminalization in Portugal," Cato Institute, 2009, 6.

23 Dianne Feinstein, Charles Schumer, and Sheldon Whitehouse, *Halting U.S. Firearms Trafficking to Mexico* (report to the U.S. Senate Caucus on International Narcotics Control, June 2011), 4.

24 "Under the Volcano," 30.

25 Luis de la Torre, "Drug Trafficking and Police Corruption" (thesis, Naval Postgraduate School, April 2008), 96.

26 Danelo, "The Many Faces of Mexico," 174.

27 Wesley Skogan and George Atunes, "Information, Apprehension, and Deterrence: Exploring the Limits of Police Productivity," in *What Works in Policing*, ed. David Bayley (Oxford: Oxford University Press, 2008), 108.

28 Dilshika Jayamaha, Scott Brady, Ben Fitzgerald, and Jason Fritz, *Lessons Learned from U.S. Government Law Enforcement in International Operations* (Carlisle Barracks, PA: Peacekeeping and Stability Operations Institute, 2010), 45–46.

29 Schroeder, "Mexico's Youngest Assassins," 29.

30 William Booth and Nick Miroff, "Mexico's Drug Lords Fall, but War Goes On," *Washington Post*, March 31, 2011, http://www.washingtonpost.com/world/mexicos -drug-lords-fall-but-war-goes-on/2011/03/28/AFn8ufAC_story.html.

31 Ibid.

32 Brands, *Mexico's Narco-Insurgency*, 39–40.

33 Francis Fukuyama and Seth Colby, "Half a Miracle," *Foreign Policy* (May/June 2011), http://www.foreignpolicy.com/articles/2011/04/25/half_a_miracle.

34 Friman, "Drug Markets and the Selective Use of Violence," 286.

35 Kenney, *From Pablo to Osama*, 216.

BIBLIOGRAPHY

Agren, David. "Oil: The Mexican Cartels' Other Deadly Business." *Toronto Globe and Mail*. December 21, 2010. http://www.theglobeandmail.com/news/world/americas/oil-the-mexican-cartels-other-deadly-business/article1845378/.

Aguilar, Ruben and Jorge Castaneda. *El Narco: La Guerra Fallida*. Mexico, DF: Punto de Lectura, 2009.

Andreas, Peter. *Border Games*. Ithaca, NY: Cornell University Press, 2009.

Arabit, Joseph M. "Violence along the Southwest Border." Statement before the House Appropriations Committee, Subcommittee on Commerce, Justice, Science, and Related Agencies, March 24, 2009. http://www.usdoj.gov/dea/speeches/s032409.pdf.

Archibold, Randal. "Hired by Customs, but Working for Mexican Cartels." *New York Times*, December 17, 2009. http://www.nytimes.com/2009/12/18/us/18corrupt.html?pagewanted=all.

———. "Mexican Prosecutors Train in U.S. for Changes in Their Legal System." *New York Times*, April 24, 2009. http://www.nytimes.com/2009/04/25/us/25prosecute.html.

Arlacchi, Pino. "The Dynamics of Illegal Markets." In *Combating Transnational Crime*, edited by Phil Williams and Dimitri Vlassis. Portland, OR: Frank Cass, 2001.

Arquilla, John, and David Ronfeldt, eds. *Networks and Netwars*. Santa Monica, CA: Rand, 2001.

Astorga, Luis. "Drug Trafficking in Mexico: A First General Assessment." UNESCO Discussion Paper No. 36.

Bayley, David, and Robert Perito. *The Police in War*. Boulder, CO: Lynne Rienner, 2010.

———. *Changing the Guard*. New York: Oxford University Press, 2006.

Beaubien, Jason. "In Just One Year, A Mexican City Turns Violent." National Public Radio, October 16, 2010. http://www.npr.org/templates/story/story.php?storyId=130592600.

———. "Saint or Sinner?" National Public Radio, April 13, 2009.

Beith, Malcolm. "Are Mexico's Drug Cartels Terrorist Groups?" Slate.com, April 15, 2010. http://www.slate.com/toolbar.aspx?action=print&id=2250990.

Bergman, Marcelo. "Creating New Soldiers in Mexico's Drug War." Foreignpolicy.com, May 17, 2010. www.foreignpolicy.com/articles/2010/05/17/creating_new_soldiers _in_mexico_s_drug_war.html.

Bonner, Robert. "New Cocaine Cowboys." *Foreign Affairs* (July/August 2010).

Booth, William, and Nick Miroff. "Mexican Cartels Send Messages of Death." msnbc.com, December 4, 2008. www.msnbc.com/id/2804515/print/1/displaymode/1098.

———. "Mexican Pirates Attack Texas Fishermen on Falcon Lake, Which Straddles Border." *Washington Post*, May 30, 2010.

———. "Traffickers along U.S.-Mexico Border Turn to Disguises." *Washington Post*, August 31, 2010.

Borger, Julian and Jo Tuckman. "Blood Brothers." *London Guardian*, March 15, 2002. http://www.guardian.co.uk/world/2002/mar/15/mexico.julianborger.

Brands, Hal. *Crime, Violence, and the Crisis in Guatemala*. Carlisle Barracks, PA: Strategic Studies Institute, 2010.

———. "Los Zetas and Mexico's Transnational Drug War." *World Policy Review*, December 29, 2009. http://www.worldpoliticsreview.com/articles/4866/los-zetas-and -mexicos-transnational-drug-war.

———. *Mexico's Narco-Insurgency and U.S. Counterdrug Policy*. Carlisle Barracks, PA: Strategic Studies Institute, May 2009.

Bruneau, Thomas. "The Maras and National Security in Central America." *Strategic Insights* (May 2005).

Bunker, Pamela, Lisa Campbell, and Robert Bunker. "Torture, Beheadings, and Narcocultos." *Small Wars and Insurgencies* (March 2010).

Bunker, Robert. "Strategic Threat: Narcos and Narcotics Overview." *Small Wars and Insurgencies* (March 2010).

Burnett, John, Marisa Peñaloza, and Robert Benincasa. "Mexico Seems to Favor Sinaloa Cartel in Drug War." National Public Radio, July 24, 2010.

Burton, Fred, and Scott Stewart. "Mexican Cartels and the Fallout from Phoenix." Stratfor, July 2, 2008. www.stratfor.com/weekly/mexican_cartels_and_fallout_phoenix.

Caldwell, Alicia. "U.S. Official: Mexican Car Bomb Likely Used Tovex." *Washington Post*, July 19, 2010. http://www.washingtonpost.com/wp-dyn/content/article/2010/07 /19/AR2010071901027.html.

Campbell, D. E. "A Saint for Lost Souls." *Foreign Policy* (May/June 2010).

Campbell, Lisa. "Los Zetas: An Operational Assessment." *Small Wars and Insurgencies* (March 2010).

Carchado, Alfredo. "Drug War Clashes between Gulf Cartel and Zetas May Escalate." *Dallas Morning News*, March 1, 2010. http://www.dallasnews.com/sharedcontent /dws/dn/latestnews/stories/030110dnintdrugwar.416aff8.html.

Carpenter, Ted Galen. "Mexico Is Becoming the Next Colombia." CATO Institute Foreign Policy Briefing no. 87, November 15, 2005.

Casey, Nicholas. "Mexico under Seige." *Wall Street Journal*, August 19, 2010. http://online.wsj.com/article/SB10001424052748704557704575437762646209270.html.

Casey, Nicholas, and James Hagerty. "Companies Shun Violent Mexico." *Wall Street Journal*, December 17, 2010. http://online.wsj.com/article /SB10001424052748703395204576023811983098994.html?mod=WSJ _hp_MIDDLENexttoWhatsNewsTop.

Casey, Nicholas, and Jose de Cordoba, "Northern Mexico's State of Anarchy." *Wall Street Journal*, November 20–21, 2010.

Cattan, Nacha. "Fed Up with Plague of Kidnappings, Mexicans Turn to Mob Justice." *Christian Science Monitor*, September 22, 2010. http://www.csmonitor.com/World /Americas/2010/0922/Fed-up-with-plague-of-kidnappings-Mexicans-turn-to-mob -justice.

———. "UN Questions Mexican Army's Role in Drug War." *Christian Science Monitor*, April 1, 2011. http://www.csmonitor.com/World/Americas/2011/0401/UN-questions -Mexican-Army-s-role-in-drug-war.

Chardy, Alfonso. "Mexicans Caught in Drug War Get U.S. Asylum." AZcentral.com, April 5, 2010.

Cohen, Saul. *Geography and Politics in a Divided World*. London: Methuen, 1964.

Cordoba, Jose de, and David Luhnow. "Mexican Army Officers Detained for Cartel Payments." *Wall Street Journal*, June 15, 2009. http://online.wsj.com/article /SB124510705768916735.html.

Cronin, Audrey Kurth. "How Al Qaeda Ends." *International Security* (Summer 2006).

Cuellar, Henry. "Five Perspectives on the Merida Initiative." American Enterprise Institute, March 2008.

Danelo, David. "The Many Faces of Mexico." *Orbis* (Winter 2011).

de la Torre, Luis. "Drug Trafficking and Police Corruption." Thesis, Naval Postgraduate School, April 2008.

Dribble, Sandra. "Tijuana Violence Slows, Drops from Spotlight." *San Diego Union Tribune*, April 26, 2010.

Ellingwood, Ken. "Why Mexico Is Not the New Colombia When It Comes to Drug Cartels." *Los Angeles Times*, September 25, 2010. http://www.latimes.com/news /nationworld/world/la-fg-mexico-colombia-20100926,0,2434157.story.

Entous, Adam, and Nathan Hodge. "U.S. Sees Heightened Threat in Mexico." *Wall Street Journal*, September 10, 2010.

Fainaru, Steve, and William Booth. "Mexico Using Torture to Battle Drug Trafficker, Rights Groups Say." *Washington Post*, July 9, 2009. http://www.washingtonpost.com/wp-dyn /content/article/2009/07/08/AR2009070804197.html.

Finklea, Kristin, William Krouse, and Marc Rosenblum. *Southwest Border Violence: Issues in Identifying and Measuring Spillover Violence*. Washington, DC: Congressional Research Service, August 25, 2010.

Finnegan, William. "Silver or Lead?" *The New Yorker*, May 31, 2010.

Fisman, Raymond, and Miguel Edward. *Economic Gangsters*. Princeton, NJ: Princeton University Press, 2008.

Franzia, Manuel Roig. "Mexican Drug Cartels Make Audacious Pitch for Recruits." *Washington Post*, May 7, 2008. http://www.washingtonpost.com/wp-dyn/content/article/2008/05/06/AR2008050602566.html.

Freeman, Laurie. *State of Siege: Drug-Related Violence and Corruption in Mexico, Washington Office on Latin America Special Report*, June 2006.

Freier, Nate. *Known Unknowns: Strategic Shocks in Defense Strategy Development*. Carlisle Barracks, PA: Strategic Studies Institute, 2008.

Friman, H. Richard. "Drug Markets and Selective Use of Violence." *Crime, Law, and Social Change* (September 2009).

———. "Forging the Vacancy Chain." *Crime, Law, and Social Change* (December 2004).

Gambetta, Diego. *Codes of the Underworld*. Princeton, NJ: Princeton University Press, 2009.

———. *The Sicilian Mafia*. Cambridge, MA: Harvard University Press, 1993.

Gienger, Viola. "Mexico, U.S. Expand Drug War beyond Military to Social Efforts." *Bloomberg Business Week*, March 24, 2010. http://www.businessweek.com/news/2010-03-24/mexico-u-s-expand-drug-war-beyond-military-to-social-efforts.html.

Ginsburg, Susan. *Security Human Mobility in an Age of Risk*. Washington, DC: Migration Policy Institute, 2010.

Godson, Roy. "Political-Criminal Nexus: Overview" In *Menace to Society*, edited by Roy Godson. New Brunswick, NJ: Transaction Publishers, 2003.

Gomez, Francisco. "Indagan Red De Mafia Japonesa en Mexico." *El Universal*, December 5, 2010. http://www.eluniversal.com.mx/nacion/182273.html.

Gomora, Doris. "Carteles Mexicanos Compran Droga en Afghanistan, Alertan." *El Universal*, January 4, 2011. http://www.eluniversal.com.mx/notas/734815.html.

Grayson, George. "La Familia: Another Deadly Syndicate." Foreign Policy Research Institute, February 2009. http://www.fpri.org/enotes/200901.grayson.lafamilia.html.

———. *Mexico: Narco-Violence and a Failed State?* New Brunswick, NJ: Transaction Publishers, 2009.

Greenwald, Glenn. "Drug Decriminalization in Portugal." Cato Institute, 2009.

Grillo, Ioan. "Drug Dealing for Jesus: Mexico's Evangelical Narcos." *Time*, July 19, 2009. http://www.time.com/time/world/article/0,8599,1911556,00.html.

Grim, Ryan. *This Is Your Country on Drugs*. Hoboken, NJ: Wiley and Sons, 2009.

Hernandez, Daniel. "Mexico Expats Warned on Travel Home." *Los Angeles Times*, November 24, 2010.

Iliff, Laurence, and Alfredo Corchado. "Drug Violence Has Moved Into Mexico City." *Dallas Morning News*, February 8, 2008. http://www.dallasnews.com/sharedcontent/dws/news/texassouthwest/stories/DN-capital_08int.ART.North.Edition1.45119ad.html.

Jayamaha, Dilshika, Scott Brady, Ben Fitzgerald, and Jason Fritz. *Lessons Learned from U.S. Government Law Enforcement in International Operations*. Carlisle Barracks, PA: Peacekeeping and Stability Operations Institute, 2010.

Jenkins, Brian. "Mexico: Failing State?" *National Journal*, March 23, 2009. http://security .nationaljournal.com/2009/03/mexico-failing-state.php.

Jonnson, Patrik. "Falcon Lake 'Pirate' Murder: Is Beheading 'Message to the Americans'?" *Christian Science Monitor*, October 13, 2010. http://www.csmonitor.com/USA/2010 /1013/Falcon-Lake-pirate-murder-Is-beheading-message-to-the-Americans.

———. "Mistaken Identity Theory Gains Traction in Falcon Lake 'Pirate' Attack." *Christian Science Monitor*, October 15, 2010. http://www.csmonitor.com/USA/2010 /1015/Mistaken-identity-theory-gains-traction-in-Falcon-Lake-pirate-attack.

Kenney, Michael. *From Pablo to Osama*. University Park: Pennsylvania State University Press, 2007.

Killebrew, Bob, and Jennifer Bernal. "Crime Wars." Center for a New American Security, September 2010.

———. "A New Threat: The Crossover of Urban Gang Warfare and Terrorism." *National Strategy Forum Review* (Fall 2008).

Kilmer, Beau, Jonathan P. Caulkins, Brittany M. Bond, and Peter H. Reuter. "Reducing Drug Trafficking Revenues and Violence in Mexico." Rand Corporation, 2010.

Krause, Lincoln. "The Guerrillas Next Door." *Low Intensity Conflict and Law Enforcement* (Spring 1999).

Lawson, Guy. "The War Next Door." Rollingstone.com, November 13, 2008. http://www.militaryphotos.net/forums/showthread.php?145209-The-War-Next-Door.

Livesey, Bruce. "Drug Cartels and the Mexican Military." *Vancouver Sun*, July 17, 2010. http://www.vancouversun.com/news/Drug+cartels+Mexican+army/3290794 /story.html.

Llana, Sarah Miller. "Mexican Workers Send Less Cash Home from U.S." *Christian Science Monitor*, January 28, 2009. http://www.csmonitor.com/World/Americas /2009/0128/p25s20-woam.html.

———. "Setbacks in Mexico's War on Corruption." *Christian Science Monitor*, December 30, 2008. http://www.csmonitor.com/World/Americas/2008/1230/p06s02-woam.html.

Longmire, Sylvia, and John Longmire IV. "Redefining Terrorism: Why Mexican Drug Trafficking Is More Than Just Organized Crime." *Journal of Strategic Studies* (November 2008).

Luhnow, David, and Jose de Cordoba. "The Perilous State of Mexico." *Wall Street Journal*, February 21, 2009. http://online.wsj.com/article/SB123518102536038463.html.

———. "War on the Other Terror." *The Australian*, February 23, 2009.

Lupsha, Peter. "Transnational Organized Crime Versus the State." *Transnational Organized Crime* (Spring 1996).

MacCoun, Robert, and Peter Reuter. *Drug War Heresies*. Cambridge: Cambridge University Press, 2001.

Manwaring, Max. *A "New" Dynamic in the Western Hemisphere Security Environment*. Carlisle Barracks, PA: Strategic Studies Institute, September 2009.

Marosi, Richard. "A Tijuana Blood Bath." *Los Angeles Times*, October 6, 2008. http://articles.latimes.com/2008/oct/06/world/fg-arellano6.

McCaffrey, Barry. "After Action Report—Visit Mexico—5–7 December 2008."

McKinley, James, Jr. "Mexican Cartels Lure American Teens as Killers." *New York Times*, June 23, 2009. http://www.nytimes.com/2009/06/23/us/23killers.html.

———. "Suspect in Juarez Says Killers Pursued Jail Guard." *New York Times*, March 31, 2010. http://www.nytimes.com/2010/04/01/world/americas/01mexico.html.

———. "Two Sides of a Border: One Violent, One Peaceful." *New York Times*, January 22, 2009. http://www.nytimes.com/2009/01/23/us/23elpaso.html.

———. "U.S. Gun Dealers Arming Mexican Drug Cartels." *New York Times*, December 6, 2009. http://www.nytimes.com/2009/02/26/world/americas/26iht-border.4 .20459692.html.

———. "U.S. Is Arms Bazaar for Mexican Cartels." *New York Times*, February 25, 2009. http://www.nytimes.com/2009/02/26/us/26borders.html.

Medrano, Lourdes. "Border Patrol Agent Killed: Are Smugglers Becoming More Daring?" *Christian Science Monitor*, December 15, 2010. http://www.csmonitor.com/USA /2010/1215/Border-patrol-agent-killed-Are-smugglers-becoming-more-daring.

Melis, Alberto. "Foreword: A View from the Borderlands." *Small Wars and Insurgencies* (March 2010).

Millman, Jose. "Mexican Pot Gangs Infiltrate Indian Reservations in the U.S." *Wall Street Journal*, November 5, 2009. http://online.wsj.com/article/SB125736987377028727.html.

Miroff, Nick. "Mexico Hopes $270 Million in Social Spending Will Help End Juarez Drug Violence." *Washington Post*, August 12, 2010. http://www.washingtonpost.com /wp-dyn/content/article/2010/08/11/AR2010081106253.html.

Mueller, John. *Remnants of War*. Ithaca, NY: Cornell University Press, 2004.

Nagle, Luz. "Corruption of Politicians, Law Enforcement, and the Judiciary in Mexico and Complicity Across the Border." *Small Wars and Insurgencies* (March 2010).

Napoleoni, Loretta. *Modern Jihad: Tracing the Dollars behind the Terror Networks*. Sterling, VA: Pluto Press, 2003.

National Drug Intelligence Center. *Arizona: High-Intensity Drug Trafficking Area, Drug Market Analysis 2009*. March 2009.

Nava, Juan. "Mexico: Failing State or Emerging Democracy?" *Military Review* (March–April 2011).

Naylor, R. T. "Violence and Illegal Economic Activity." *Crime, Law, and Social Change* (September 2009).

Nordstrom, Carolyn. *Global Outlaws*. Los Angeles: University of California Press, 2007.

Olson, Alexandra. "Amid Drug War, Mexico Less Deadly Than a Decade Ago." *El Paso Times*, February 7, 2010. http://www.elpasotimes.com/texas/ci_14353710.

O'Neill, Shannon. "The Real War in Mexico." *Foreign Affairs* (July/August 2009).

Osorno, Diego Enrique. "Vigilante Groups Appear in Five Mexican States." *El Milenio*, January 26, 2009. http://narcosphere.narconews.com/notebook/kristin-bricker /2009/01/vigilante-groups-appear-five-mexican-states.

Paoli, Letizia. "Criminal Fraternities or Criminal Enterprises?" In *Combating Transnational Crime*, edited by Phil Williams and Dimitri Vlassis. Portland, OR: Frank Cass, 2001.

Payan, Tony. *The Three U.S.-Mexico Border Wars*. Westport, CT: Praeger Security International, 2006.

Perez-Rocha, Manuel. "Mexico: Neither a Failed State nor Model." Institute for Policy Studies, February 23, 2009. http://www.ips-dc.org/articles/mexico_neither_a_failed _state_nor_a_model.

Phillips, Jen. "Mexico's New Super-Cartel Ups Violence in Power Play." *Mother Jones*, April 13, 2010. http://motherjones.com/mojo/2010/04/evolution-mexicos-cartel-war.

Potter, Mark. "Drug War 'Alarming' U.S. Officials." msnbc.com, June 25, 2008. http://worldblog.msnbc.msn.com/archive/2008/06/25/1166487.aspx.

Quinones, Sam. "State of War." *Foreign Policy* (March/April 2009).

Raab, Jorg, and H. Brinton Milward. "Dark Networks as Problems." *Journal of Public Administration Research and Theory* (October 2003).

Reuter, Peter. "Systemic Violence in Drug Markets." *Crime, Law, and Social Change* (September 2009).

Rios, Viridiana. "Mexican Assassins on the Cheap." International Relations and Security Network, October 11, 2010. http://www.isn.ethz.ch/isn/Current-Affairs/ISN -Insights/Detail?lng=en&id=122286&contextid734=122286&contextid735 =122282&tabid=122282.

Roebuck, Jeremy. "Authorities: Gulf Cartel, Zetas Gang Up on Each Other as Their Arrangement Dies." *Rio Grande Monitor*, March 10, 2010. http://www.themonitor.com /articles/gulf-36258-arrangement-reynosa.html.

Rotella, Sebastian. "Former U.S. Anti-Drug Official Arrest 'A Complete Shock.'" *Los Angeles Times*, September 17, 2009. http://articles.latimes.com/2009/sep/17/nation/na-drug -charges17.

Roth, Mitchel, and Murat Sever. "The Kurdish Workers Party (PKK) as Criminal Syndicate." *Studies in Conflict and Terrorism* (2007).

Schelling, Thomas. *Arms and Influence*. Westport, CT: Greenwood Press, 1977.

Schroeder, Jana. "Mexico's Youngest Assassins." *Homeland Security Today* (March 2011).

Seelke, Claire, and Kristin Finklea. *U.S.-Mexican Security Cooperation: The Mérida Initiative and Beyond*. Washington, DC: Congressional Research Services, 2010.

Selee, Andrew, David Shirk, and Eric Olson. "Five Myths about Mexico's Drug War." *Washington Post*, March 28, 2010.

Seper, Jerry. "Mexican Military Incursions Reported." *Washington Times*, January 17, 2006.

Sheridan, Mary Beth. "Military Broadens U.S. Push to Help Mexico Battle Drug Cartels." *Washington Post*, November 10, 2010.

Sherwell, Philip. "Mexican Drug Wars Force Police to Claim Asylum in U.S." *London Daily Telegraph*, www.telegraph.co.uk, April 11, 2009.

Shirk, David. "Justice Reform in Mexico, Working Paper Series on U.S.-Mexico Security Cooperation." Transborder Institute: University of San Diego, April 2010.

Skogan, Wesley, and George Atunes. "Information, Apprehension, and Deterrence: Exploring the Limits of Police Productivity" in *What Works in Policing,* edited by David Bayley. Oxford: Oxford University Press, 2008.

Stewart, Scott, and Alex Posey. "Mexico: The War with the Cartels in 2009." Stratfor, December 9, 2009. http://www.stratfor.com/weekly/20091209_mexico_war_cartels_2009.

Sullivan, John. "Counter-Supply and Counter-Violence Approaches to Narcotics Trafficking." *Small Wars and Insurgencies* (March 2010).

———. "Police-Military Interaction in Mexico's Drug War." *Air and Space Power Journal* (October 2009). http://www.airpower.au.af.mil/apjinternational/apj-s/2009/3tri09/sullivaneng.htm.

Turbiville, Graham, ed. *Global Dimensions of High Intensity Crime and Low Intensity Conflict.* Chicago: University of Illinois, 1995.

United Nations Special Rapporteur. *Independence of Judges and Lawyers: Report on the Mission to Mexico.* January 24, 2002.

United States Agency for International Development. *Central America and Mexico Gang Assessment.* April 2006.

United States Department of Health and Human Services, results from the 2009 National Survey on Drug Use and Health. September 2010. http://www.oas.samhsa.gov/NSDUH/2k9NSDUH/2k9ResultsP.pdf.

United States Department of Justice, *National Drug Threat Assessment 2008.* Washington, DC: National Drug Intelligence Center, 2007.

United States Immigration and Customs Enforcement. "Statement of Marcy Forman, Director." March 1, 2006. www.ice.gov/doclib/pi/news/testimony/060301homelandpdf.

United States Joint Forces Command. *Joint Operating Environment 2008.* November 25, 2008.

Varese, Federico. *The Russian Mafia.* Oxford: Oxford University, 2001.

Volkov, Vadim. *Violent Entrepreneurs.* Ithaca, NY: Cornell University Press, 2002.

Vulliamy, Ed. "Killing for Kudos." *London Guardian Online,* February 7, 2010. http://www.guardian.co.uk/world/2010/feb/07/mexico-drug-war.

Wald, Elijah. *Narcocorrido.* New York: Rayo, 2002.

Walser, Ray. "Mexico, Drug Cartels, and the Mérida Initiative." *Heritage Foundation Backgrounder,* July 23, 2008.

Weber, Paul. "U.S. Border Patrol Agents in 'Firefight' with Mexican Gang." ABC News, September 13, 2010. http://abcnews.go.com/US/wirestory?id=11627914&page=2.

Wilkinson, Tracy, and Ken Ellingwood. "Mexico's Army Failures Hamper Drug War." *Los Angeles Times,* December 29, 2010. http://articles.latimes.com/2010/dec/29/world/la-fg-mexico-army-20101230.

Williams, Phil. "Illicit Markets, Weak States, and Violence: Iraq and Mexico." *Crime, Law, and Social Change* (September 2009).

———. "The International Drug Trade." In *Global Dimensions of High-Intensity Crime and Low-Intensity Conflict,* edited by Graham Turbiville. Chicago: University of Illinois, 1995.

———. "Organizing Transnational Crime." in *Combating Transnational Crime,* edited by Phil Williams and Dimitri Vlassis. Portland, OR: Frank Cass, 2001.

———. "Transnational Criminal Organizations and International Security." In *In Athena's Camp,* edited by John Arquilla and David Ronfeldt. Santa Monica, CA: Rand Corporation, 1997.

Williams, Phil, and Dimitri Vlassis, eds. *Combating Transnational Crime.* Portland, OR: Frank Cass, 2001.

Wood, Daniel. "Robert Krentz Killing Stokes Fears of Rampant Illegal Immigration." *Christian Science Monitor,* March 31, 2010. http://www.csmonitor.com/USA/2010/0331/Robert-Krentz-killing-stokes-fears-of-rampant-illegal-immigration.

Wright, Alan. *Organised Crime.* Cullompton, UK: Willan Publishing, 2006.

INDEX

The letter g following a page number denotes a graph.

The letter m following a page number denotes a map.

The letter t following a page number denotes a table.

"accidental narco" syndrome, 19, 120, 123, 151

Arellano Félix family, 36, 37

Arellano Félix Organization, 17, 36–38

ATF (Bureau of Alcohol, Tobacco, Firearms, and Explosives), 35, 100–102, 143

Ávila Beltrán, Sandra, 34

Baja California, Mexico, 37–38, 57, 60, 96–97, 149

Baja California Sur, Mexico, 64

Barrio Azteca, 42, 87

Beltrán Leyva, Alfredo, 40, 41, 96

Beltrán Leyva, Arturo, 40, 41, 64, 96, 125

Beltrán Leyva, Carlos, 96

Beltrán Leyva, Hector, 41

BLO (Beltrán-Leyva Organization)
  alliances, 28, 40–41, 49, 61
  founders, 40
  government intervention, 49, 96
  hitmen, 79
  informants, 81
  overview, 40–41
  revenge killings, 124
  rivals, 39
  territory, 61–62

border
  crossing, 5, 71, 80
  incursions, 74
  security, 5, 74, 87, 98, 101–3, 116

Border Patrol, 36, 73–74, 79, 87, 102, 103, 135

Borsellino, Paolo, 140

"brain drain," 123–24

Bravo, Roberto, 64, 125

Buenos Aires National Wildlife Refuge, 75

Bunker, Robert, 7

Bureau of Alcohol, Tobacco, Firearms, and Explosives. *See* ATF

Calderón Administration
  policy, 91–98
  reforms, 93–95, 99, 110–11, 113, 115–17, 141, 150
  supportive neighboring governments, 110

Calderón, Felipe, 2, 3, 5, 59

Calderón, Igor, 64, 125

Cali cartel (Colombian), 11, 112, 151

Camarena, Enrique, 37

car bomb, 42

Caribbean smuggling routes, 4, 115

Cártel de Jalisco Nueva Generación, 49

cartelitos, 116

Cartel Pacifico Sur faction, 41

cartels
  alliances, 16, 48–51, 61–62, 65, 120, 122
  and al Qaeda, 85–86
  balance of power, 20, 120–23
  community support or acquiescence, 31–32, 44
  compared to Colombian cartels, 7, 8, 11, 13, 18
  corporate logic, 25–32
  countercartel strategy, 141, 147–51
  gang involvement, 23, 30–31, 36–47, 84–85
  goals, 25, 55
  group cohesion and identity, 30–31
  hypercompetitive markets, 13–17, 19–20
  illegal migrant smuggling, 26, 80
  information operations, 51
  major players, 18, 36–47
  manipulation of prisons, 99
  and the media, 27, 47, 51

ABOUT THE AUTHOR

Paul Rexton Kan is associate professor of national security studies and the Henry L. Stimson Chair of Military Studies at the U.S. Army War College. He is the author of the book *Drugs and Contemporary Warfare* (Potomac Books, 2009) and numerous articles on the intersection of drug trafficking, crime, and modern forms of armed conflict. He has also served as the senior visiting counternarcotics adviser at NATO Headquarters in Kabul, Afghanistan, and has provided advice to the U.S. Office of National Drug Control Policy. He lives in Carlisle, Pennsylvania.

www.ingramcontent.com/pod-product-compliance
Lightning Source LLC
Chambersburg PA
CBHW021154160426
42812CB00082B/3085/J